Hospital-Sector Inflation

Hospital-Sector Inflation

David S. Salkever
The Johns Hopkins University

LexingtonBooks
D.C. Heath and Company
Lexington, Massachusetts
Toronto

Library of Congress Cataloging in Publication Data

Salkever, David S
    Hospital-sector inflation.

    Includes bibliographical references and index.
    1.   Hospitals—United States—Cost of operation.
2. Inflation (Finance)—United States. 3. Hospitals—United States—
Rates. I.   Title.
RA981.A2S18   338.4′3   76-11340
ISBN 0-669-00704-8

Published simultaneously in Canada.

Printed in the United States of America.

International Standard Book Number: 0-669-00704-8

Library of Congress Catalog Card Number: 76-11340

Contents

List of Tables

Acknowledgments

Since the work on this volume spanned ten years and several locations, there are many organizations and individuals to whom I am indebted for their assistance. Chapter 1 was originally part of my doctoral thesis. In this effort, I benefited tremendously from the guidance of my thesis committee, Professors Martin Feldstein, John Dunlop, and Rashi Fein, and from the helpful comments of Jan Acton and Ralph Berry. Chapter 2 originally appeared in the *Journal of Political Economy* (Vol. 80, 1972, pp. 1144–1166). Thanks are due to the University of Chicago Press for permission to reprint this paper. Martin Feldstein and William Raduchel provided valuable advice and suggestions during the course of the research, Victor Fuchs, Joseph Newhouse, and a journal referee also offered several helpful comments.

The hospital cost data used in chapters 1 and 2 were provided by the Associated Hospital Service of New York. For substantial assistance in my efforts to collect and interpret the data, I am grateful to James Ingram, Ed Cooney, Larry Cafasso, and Nathan Morrison. Financial support at Harvard University for work on chapters 1 and 2 was provided by U.S. Public Health Service Training Grant CH-00008-03 and by a grant from the Carnegie Foundation.

A short version of chapter 3 appeared in the *Quarterly Review of Economics and Business* (Vol. 15, 1975, pp. 33–48). I wish to thank the Bureau of Economic and Business Research of the University of Illinois for permission to reprint this paper. Support from the National Center for Health Services Research under Grant 5R01 HS 0110 is gratefully acknowledged.

In preparing chapter 4, I benefited from access to several unpublished works. I am especially grateful to Pat O'Donoghue of Spectrum Research for providing a copy of Spectrum's Indiana report and to Bob Helms of the American Enterprise Institute for providing a manuscript copy of a forthcoming book by Paul Ginsburg.

There are, of course, many other persons who helped the work along in various ways. Limitations of space (and memory) preclude me from listing them here, though my gratitude for their assistance is nonetheless sincere.

Finally, I dedicate this book to my parents who, for more years than they care to remember, nurtured my scholarly inclinations with just the right mix of enthusiastic praise and (usually) restrained criticism.

Introduction

The four chapters in this volume focus on the empirical analysis of hospital cost inflation. Since they were completed over a ten-year period, their subject matter reflects the changing emphases of hospital economics over this time span. Yet I believe that all the chapters are still relevant to current health policy research.

The first chapter is an exercise in cost-inflation accounting. During the 1960s one of the justifications of rising hospital costs commonly offered by medical practitioners and hospital executives was that higher costs reflected a change in the hospital's product mix. The cases being treated were more complex, the volume of outpatient services was increasing rapidly, the volume of educational services was increasing rapidly, and the treatments provided to patients were becoming more and more sophisticated. This chapter attempts to measure the contributions of these four types of product-mix changes to observed cost inflation. Because of limitations in the data and methods employed, most of the findings relate specifically to the first three types of product-mix change. Using data from short-term general hospitals in southeastern New York State for the 1961–1964 period, I found that these three types account for only about one-tenth of the actual increase in average cost per case. The conclusion is that the large increases in average cost per case over this period reflect other inflationary factors, such as increased technical sophistication or intensity of treatment, and higher input prices.

Another issue examined in chapter 1 is the effect on hospital costs of medical education. The analysis indicates that medical education activities of hospitals substantially increase their costs per case, primarily because of longer average lengths of stay in teaching hospitals.

For several reasons the precise quantitative findings of the study are of limited applicability at this time. The product-mix data employed (especially the data on inpatient case mix) are rather crude, and the omission of the cost of private attending physicians for nonteaching hospitals imparts an upward bias to the estimated cost impact of medical education. The current significance of these findings is further diminished by the age of the data and by the fact that a number of more recent studies based on better data are now available.[1] However, chapter 1 devotes considerable attention to methodological issues, such as the specification of hospital cost functions and the potential problem of simultaneous equation bias. For this reason I hope that the chapter will be of methodologic interest to other researchers in the field.

The issues addressed in chapter 1 are still high on the agenda of the academics and policymakers who are attempting to design and implement prospective rate-setting systems for hospitals. Considerable effort is now being devoted to developing methods of adjusting prospective rates for interhospital differences and intertemporal changes in product mix. Prospective rate setting also highlights the need to determine the additional cost to the hospital of clinical education programs and to assign responsibility for this cost among groups of patients and the community at large.

In the second and third chapters the primary concern is the influence of forces outside the hospital industry on rising hospital costs and wages. The second chapter was originally conceived as an extension of Martin Feldstein's seminal work on the rising demand for hospital services.[2] Feldstein constructed a model in which the rising cost of hospital care was assumed to be due solely to rising demand.[3] In this chapter, I allow for the possibility that rising costs are due to both rising demand and factor-market conditions.

The most important methodological feature of this second chapter, and of Feldstein's earlier study, is the use of a behavioral model that depicts the hospital as choosing its cost level subject to market and technological constraints. All previous econometric work on hospital costs had taken a technological (or quasi-technological) approach. But the behavioral approach is more appropriate for assessing the underlying causes of cost inflation and the effectiveness of policies to curb inflation. For this reason it has been applied in a number of more recent studies.[4]

The third chapter further explores the possibility that factor-market conditions that were omitted from Feldstein's original model in fact played a role in cost inflation. More specifically, it examines the influence of changing product-demand and labor-market conditions on the wages of unskilled female hospital workers during the 1960s. The analysis is based on data for large metropolitan areas from the U.S. Bureau of Labor Statistics' hospital industry wage surveys.

Results from chapters 2 and 3 indicate that while rising demand was an important cause of cost inflation, changing factor-market conditions also played a role in the inflationary process during the 1960s. Subsequent studies have confirmed this finding.[5] But studies based on more recent data suggest that increases in demand (generated by increasing insurance coverage), which were substantial during the 1960s, may no longer be an important cause of rising costs.[6]

The fourth chapter reviews recent econometric research concerning the effects of rate-setting programs on hospital costs. The principal concern is programs operating in individual states, although findings from recent studies of the federal Economic Stabilization Program are also briefly reviewed. One purpose of this chapter is to present in some detail the results from these studies (some of which are not yet widely available) and to discuss the possible interpretations of the results. A second and perhaps more important purpose is to critically review the methods used in these studies. I hope that this discussion will be of interest to other investigators undertaking further research in the field of hospital regulation.

Notes

1. On the effects of medical education on costs, see Adele P. Massell and James R. Hosek, *Estimating the Effects of Teaching on the Costs of Inpatient Care: The Case of Radiology Treatments*, Rand Corporation Report R-1751-HEW (Santa Monica, Ca., August 1975); and the references cited therein. A number of recent studies have analyzed the effect of product mix (or case mix) on costs in the cross-sectional framework. For references see Judith R. Lave and Lester B. Lave, "Hospital Cost Functions," in *Health Handbook* ed. George Chacko (Amsterdam: North Holland, 1976). However, to my knowledge, more recent work on the cost implications of changes in product mix over time has been limited.

2. Martin S. Feldstein, "Hospital Cost Inflation: A Study in Non-profit Price Dynamics," *American Economic Review* 61 (December 1971): 853–872.

3. In this model the cost (and price) of a day of hospital care was determined in the short run by the level of demand, the available stock of beds, and the hospital's desired occupancy rate. Rising wages were only assumed to influence cost in the long run by affecting the hospital's desired stock of beds. However, this long-run relationship was not included in Feldstein's empirical model.

4. See Lave and Lave, "Hospital Cost Functions," for several references.

5. Carol M. McCarthy, "Supply and Demand and Hospital Cost Inflation," *Medical Care Review* 33(August 1976): 923–248.

6. Joseph P. Newhouse, *The Erosion of the Medical Marketplace, or What the Market Hath Joined Together, Let Not Health Insurance Put Asunder*. Rand Corporation Report R-2141-HEW (Santa Monica, Ca., May 1977).

1 A Study of the Impact of Product-Mix Change on Hospital Cost Inflation

Various explanations have been offered for the rapid rise in hospital costs, including the catching up of hospital wages, rising demand, and the changing nature of the hospital's product.[1] Using the conventional measures of average cost per inpatient-day or per inpatient case, we can identify four types of change in hospital output that might account for increases in average cost: increases in the volume of outpatient services, increases in the volume of educational services, increases in the complexity of the inpatient cases for which treatment was provided, and increases in the sophistication of treatment techniques.[2]

This chapter assesses the quantitative importance of these product-mix changes by using regression analysis to obtain a quasi-technological relationship between product mix and average cost. This relationship is used to predict the changes in cost that would have taken place without product-mix change. The difference between these estimated changes and the observed changes in cost gives a quantitative estimate of the impact of product-mix change on cost inflation. The estimate of the change in cost that would have occurred without product-mix change is a meaningful measure of inflation in cost per unit of output, because it applies to a specifically defined composite product.

I shall attempt to estimate the impact of product-mix change on inflation in seventy-three short-term general hospitals in southeastern New York State over the period 1961–1964. The first section discusses the methodology of this attempt. The second section presents the measures of product mix used in the study. The quasi-technological relationship between product mix and cost is simply a statistical cost function. This function was estimated cross-sectionally from 1964 data, and the third section reports the results of the estimation process. The fourth section presents my estimates of the impacts on inflation of product-mix changes of various kinds and discusses the implications of these estimates. Appendix A to this chapter reports some further results. Appendix B provides a more complete description of the sample of hospitals and gives information on data sources, definitions, and adjustments.

Methodology

The first task is to estimate a relationship between average cost and product mix for the year 1964. This relationship will be of the general form:

1

$$AC_{i64} = F_{64}(U_{i64}, S_{i64}, p_{1i64}, \ldots, p_{ni64}, u_{i64}) \qquad (1.1)$$

where AC is average cost, U is a measure of the intensity of capital utilization, S is a measure of size, p_j is the jth measure of product mix, u is an error term, the subscript 64 refers to the year 1964, and the subscript i refers to the ith hospital.

This estimated relationship will then be used to obtain $\overline{AC}_{i64}$, which is my estimate of what observed average cost in the ith hospital in 1964 would have been if its product mix in 1964 had been the same as in 1961. $\overline{AC}_{i64}$ is defined by

$$\overline{AC}_{i64} = F_{64}(U_{i64}, S_{i64}, p_{1i61}, \ldots, p_{ni61}, u_{i64}) \qquad (1.2)$$

where p_{ji61} is the ith hospital's jth measure of product mix for the year 1961.[3]

The quantity $(\overline{AC}_{i64}/AC_{i61}) - 1$ is the estimate of the rate of increase, in the ith hospital, of the average cost of producing the composite product defined by $(p_{1i61}, \ldots, p_{ni61})$. The difference between this rate and the observed rate of increase of average costs, $(AC_{i64}/AC_{i61}) - 1$, is the estimate of the impact of product-mix change on cost inflation in the ith hospital. This quantity is equal to $(AC_{i64} - \overline{AC}_{i64})/AC_{i61}$.

The method just described is not the only way to obtain a meaningful measure of inflation for the ith hospital and an estimate of the impact of product-mix change on observed inflation. For example, we might instead estimate a cross-sectional cost function for 1961 and thereby obtain

$$\overline{AC}_{i61} = F_{61}(U_{i61}, S_{i61}, p_{1i64}, \ldots, p_{ni64}, u_{i61})$$

Then $(AC_{i64}/\overline{AC}_{i61}) - 1$ would be the estimate of the rate of increase, in the ith hospital, of the average cost of producing the composite product defined by $(p_{1i64}, \ldots, p_{ni64})$, and $(AC_{i64}/AC_{i61}) - (AC_{i64}/\overline{AC}_{i61})$ would be the estimate of product-mix change on cost inflation in the ith hospital.

Both methods decompose observed inflation into inflation for a specific composite product and inflation due to changes in this product (product-mix change). That these methods yield different results is a reflection of the index-number problem. In other words, in defining a rate of cost inflation for a composite product, we must choose a set of weights by which this product is defined. Thus $(p_{1i61}, \ldots, p_{ni61})$ $(p_{1i64}, \ldots, p_{ni64})$ are two sets of weights that might be chosen. The nature of the index-number problem implies that the choice between these two sets of weights is arbitrary. I shall choose the former set, but this arbitrary choice will affect the results.[4]

Measurement of Output and Product Mix

The assumption that the composite product of each hospital can be described by n product-mix measures is equivalent to the assumption that each hospital produces $n + 1$ products, with the output of each product denoted by $Q_k, k = 1, \ldots, n + 1$. They are equivalent because one of the Q_k's may be chosen to represent the level of output in the hospital and the remaining Q_k's may be divided by this level, thereby yielding the p_j's of the preceding section. This section first considers the problem of choosing the Q_k that is the most appropriate measure of the level of output and then presents the product-mix measures (p_j's) used in the analysis.

Measuring the Level of Output

If the estimated cost functions did not contain only one measure of capacity utilization, we could arbitrarily choose any one of the Q_k's as the measure of the level of output. But since we use only one measure of capacity utilization, this measure obviously should be the ratio of the level of inpatient care to the capacity to provide such care.[5] Thus the level of output should be measured by the level of inpatient care.[6] But how should the latter be defined?

I have chosen to define the level of inpatient care as the number of cases treated (measured by the number of discharges; including deaths but excluding newborn children). Thus the case is the basic unit of output for the product inpatient care. The case was chosen rather than the inpatient-day because of the potentially perverse behavior of cost per patient-day as a measure of the level of hospital costs. If, for example, a more economical use of hospital resources were achieved by shortening lengths of stay, cost per patient-day would increase. This would imply the odd conclusion that such a more economical use of hospital resources was inflationary.[7]

On the other hand, a number of recent studies of hospital costs have used the inpatient-day rather than the case as the basic unit of output.[8] This practice may be justified on the ground that case-mix data were not available for these studies. If interhospital variation in case-mix affects interhospital variation in cost per case primarily through variations in length of stay, the omission of case-mix variables from estimated cross-sectional average cost functions will probably result in more seriously biased coefficient estimates if the dependent variable is cost per case than if it is cost per day.[9] Case-mix data were available for this study, however, and thus case-mix variables were included directly in cross-sectional regressions of average cost per case.

Measurement of Product Mix

The hospitals under study produce three types of product: inpatient care, ambulatory patient care, and education.[10] While the level of output of inpatient care is measured by the total number of cases, we shall also distinguish among inpatient cases according to case type. For example, with m different case types each hospital's output of inpatient care will be represented by the total number of cases, denoted by Q, and by m product-mix measures of the form Q_j/Q, where Q_j is the number of cases of type j.

The case-mix data used in this study consist of a three-way break-down of total patient load in the same hospitals: by sex, by age, and by diagnostic category.[11] The data were gathered in two one-day censuses of all inpatients on October 20, 1964, and May 10, 1961.[12] Table 1–1 presents the means and standard deviations for the patient categories.[13]

Since there are twenty-nine separate categories and only about seventy hospitals in this sample, the inclusion of all the case-mix information in the cross-sectional average cost regressions would be extremely expensive in terms of degrees of freedom. I therefore decided to use a principal components analysis to obtain a smaller number of case-mix variables that would still contain a substantial amount of the information given by all the individual case types.

The results of the principal components analysis are presented in table 1–2.[14] Each principal component is defined as a linear combination of the original case-mix variables.[15] The jth principal component C_j is thus defined as $\Sigma_i a_{ji} c_i$, where the a_{ji}'s are the coefficients listed in the jth column of table 1–2 and where the c_i's are the corresponding original case-mix variables.[16] Since the original case-mix variables were all expressed as percentages, the principal components were extracted from the variance-covariance matrix of these variables rather than from their correlation matrix.[17]

By adding the percentages in the first row of table 1–2, we see that the first seven principal components explain 82 percent of the total case-mix variance across hospitals. This indicates that the seven components provide a good summary of the information contained in the original variables. Since the components are used only to provide this summary, there is no reason to try to "identify" them.[18] Furthermore, an examination of the correlations between the components and the case-mix variables, given in table 1–3, indicates that such identification would be difficult.[19] Table 1–4 lists, for each component, the five case-mix variables with the largest (positive or negative) correlations and shows that the first component may be interpreted either as an index of the absence of obstetrical activity or as an index of the presence of older patients with circulatory

Table 1–1
Means and Standard Deviations of Case-Mix Categories

	1961		1964	
Category	Mean	Standard Deviation	Mean	Standard Deviation
Male	40.20	8.03	41.70	7.68
12 years old and under	9.84	5.32	8.77	5.12
13 to 19 years	3.56	2.23	4.27	2.35
20 to 34 years	18.55	6.74	16.02	6.10
35 to 49 years	18.23	5.35	17.18	5.47
50 to 64 years	22.52	6.90	23.93	6.93
Age not available	1.72	5.81	1.45	2.46
Infective and parasitic diseases	1.10	1.35	1.06	1.05
Malignant neoplasms	5.57	3.42	7.55	3.76
Benign and unspecified neoplasms	5.40	3.17	3.85	2.45
Allergic and metabolic diseases	2.84	1.82	2.70	2.35
Diseases of the blood	0.53	0.70	0.68	0.84
Mental disorders	0.27	0.80	0.61	1.32
Nervous system diseases	4.26	2.59	5.20	3.73
Circulatory system diseases	14.42	5.49	15.68	5.62
Respiratory system diseases	9.22	4.88	8.16	4.48
Digestive system diseases	16.75	4.55	16.58	4.46
Genitourinary system diseases	8.15	3.36	8.50	3.46
Obstetrical care	12.74	7.27	9.63	6.62
Skin and cellular system diseases	1.80	2.10	1.34	1.28
Bone diseases	2.91	1.99	3.27	2.28
Congenital malformations	0.37	0.56	0.66	0.88
Certain diseases of early infancy	0.12	0.35	0.20	0.49
Symptoms, senility, and ill-defined	2.40	1.80	1.31	1.15
Accidents, poisonings, and violence	10.07	4.68	11.83	6.44
Special conditions and examinations	0.33	1.46	0.19	0.99
Female[a]	59.80	—	58.30	—
65 years old and over[a]	25.58	—	28.38	—
Premature births[a]	0.75	—	1.00	—

Note: All numbers are expressed as percentages of total inpatients, excluding normal newborn children.

[a]This category was not included in the principal components analysis.

disorders. The second component seems to indicate the extent of pediatric activity.[20] The fifth component might be interpreted as an indicator of the absence of patients with neoplasms.[21]

These "identifications" are anything but clear-cut. Examination of table 1–3 reveals that numerous case-mix variables were correlated almost as strongly with one or more of the seven components as the variables listed in table 1–4. If these other variables are also considered, the problem of identification seems impossible.[22]

The seven principal components obtained from the original case-mix variables will be used as measures of inpatient product mix.

Table 1–2
Definitions of Principal Components and Percentages of Case-Mix Variation Explained by Each

	Component						
	1	2	3	4	5	6	7
Percentage of Case-Mix Variance	30.8	18.2	10.0	7.1	7.0	5.5	3.8
Coefficient							
Male	.4768	.3546	.3881	-.1423	.2256	-.4294	.3883
12 years old and under	-.1804	.3765	-.1011	.1228	.0964	-.2732	-.2946
13 to 19 years	-.0209	.1335	.0116	-.0532	-.0474	.0680	.0104
20 to 34 years	-.4498	-.0209	.1046	.2121	.3926	-.1103	.0638
35 to 49 years	-.0805	.1253	.5438	-.4333	-.4018	.0447	-.3088
50 to 64 years	.4104	-.3660	.2783	.4272	.1706	-.0247	-.0772
Age not available	.0178	.0392	-.0373	-.1286	.0450	.0525	.0103
Infective and parasitic diseases	.0199	-.0056	.0050	-.0027	-.0324	.0153	.0260
Malignant neoplasms	-.0891	-.1177	.0576	.1187	-.3557	-.0752	.2781
Benign and unspecified neoplasms	-.0417	-.0754	.0993	-.0693	-.1581	.0249	.0143
Allergic and metabolic diseases	.0614	-.0542	.0909	-.0057	.0876	-.0934	-.0135
Diseases of the blood	.0161	-.0038	-.0095	-.0256	.0160	-.0422	-.0347
Mental disorders	.0276	.0069	.0554	-.0230	-.0166	-.0135	-.0310
Nervous system diseases	.0200	-.0877	-.3354	-.1801	-.1204	.0561	.4491
Circulatory system diseases	.2908	-.2766	-.2415	-.5011	.4039	.0443	-.3532
Respiratory system diseases	.0796	.1941	-.2697	.2686	-.1500	-.4260	-.3424
Digestive system diseases	.0821	-.0394	.2938	.3351	.0378	.4634	-.1756
Gentiourinary system diseases	-.0644	-.1159	.0805	.0043	-.1564	-.2550	-.2154
Obstetrical care	-.4808	-.0743	.2823	-.1578	.3899	-.0711	.1271
Skin and cellular system diseases	.0151	.0149	.0503	.0655	.0058	-.0420	.0485
Bone diseases	.0334	-.0349	-.0342	.0916	-.1591	-.0018	.1800
Congenital malformations	-.0083	-.0070	.0121	.0171	-.0017	.0025	-.0150
Certain diseases of early infancy	-.0042	.0039	.0010	.0011	.0013	.0047	-.0065
Symptoms, senility, and ill-defined	-.0165	.0205	-.0378	.0099	.0585	-.0267	.0612
Accidents, poisonings, and violence	.1105	.6288	-.0776	.0591	.1526	.4749	.0099
Special conditions and examinations	-.0029	-.0172	-.0397	-.0232	-.0062	-.0409	-.0170

Table 1–3
Correlations of Case-Mix Variables with Components

Case-Mix Variable	Component						
	1	2	3	4	5	6	7
Male	.727	.415	.336	−.104	.163	−.276	.207
12 years old and under	−.402	.644	−.128	.132	.102	−.257	−.229
13 to 19 years	−.102	.510	.032	−.125	−.110	.141	.018
20 to 34 years	−.823	−.029	.109	.186	.342	−.085	.041
35 to 49 years	−.172	.206	.661	−.445	−.409	.040	−.231
50 to 64 years	.694	−.475	.267	.347	.137	−.018	−.046
Age not available	.083	.142	−.100	−.291	.101	.104	.017
Infective and parasitic diseases	.200	−.043	.028	−.013	−.154	.065	.091
Malignant neoplasms	−.275	−.279	.101	.176	−.523	−.098	.300
Benign and unspecified neoplasms	−.200	−.277	.270	−.160	−.360	.050	.024
Allergic and metabolic diseases	.307	−.208	.258	−.014	.208	−.197	.024
Diseases of the blood	.223	−.040	−.075	−.171	.106	−.247	−.168
Mental disorders	.244	.047	.278	−.098	−.070	−.050	−.096
Nervous system diseases	.062	−.210	−.594	−.269	−.178	.074	.488
Circulatory system diseases	.554	−.405	−.262	−.459	.366	.036	−.235
Respiratory system diseases	.207	.388	−.399	.336	−.185	−.468	−.311
Digestive system diseases	.212	−.078	.432	.417	.046	.506	−.159
Genitourinary system diseases	−.217	−.300	.154	.007	−.251	−.363	−.254
Obstetrical care	−.833	−.099	.278	−.132	.321	−.052	.077
Skin and cellulary system diseases	.137	.104	.259	.285	.025	−.161	.154
Bone diseases	.169	−.136	−.098	.223	−.383	−.004	.318
Congenital malformations	−.111	−.072	.092	.110	−.011	.127	−.070
Certain diseases of early infancy	−.101	.071	.130	.012	.015	.048	−.054
Symptoms, senility, and ill-defined	−.168	.159	−.218	.048	.282	−.114	.217
Accidents, poisonings, and violence	.196	.857	−.078	.050	.129	.356	.006
Special conditions and examinations	−.033	−.150	−.256	−.127	−.033	−.196	−.068

Each hospital's output of ambulatory patient care was measured by total annual ambulatory patient visits. This total includes visits to emergency rooms and outpatient clinics and visits by patients referred to the hospital by private physicians.[23] It may seem desirable, a priori, to distinguish among these three types of visit, especially between emergency room visits and the other two types.[24] This was not done, however, for two reasons. First, the modest size of the sample of hospitals indicated that the information gained by disaggregating ambulatory visits would not be sufficient to justify the resulting loss in degrees of freedom. Second, there is often little or no distinction between the kinds of care rendered to emergency room patients and that rendered to other patients.[25]

Educational output was divided into two components: nurse education and physician education. (No data were available on education of other types of health professionals.) The number of student nurses in the

Table 1–4
Case-Mix Categories Most Closely Correlated with Components

Component 1		*Component 5*	
Obstetrical care	(−)	Malignant neoplasms	(−)
20 to 34 years	(−)	35 to 49 years	(−)
Male	(+)	Bone diseases	(−)
50 to 64 years	(+)	Circulatory system diseases	(+)
Circulatory system diseases	(+)	Benign and unspecified neoplasms	(−)
Component 2		*Component 6*	
Accidents	(+)	Digestive system diseases	(+)
12 years and under	(+)	Respiratory system diseases	(−)
13 to 19 years	(+)	Genitourinary system diseases	(−)
50 to 64 years	(−)	Accidents	(+)
Male	(+)	Male	(−)
Component 3		*Component 7*	
35 to 49 years	(+)	Nervous system diseases	(+)
Nervous system diseases	(−)	Bone diseases	(+)
Digestive system diseases	(+)	Respiratory system diseases	(−)
Respiratory system diseases	(−)	Malignant neoplasms	(+)
Male	(+)	Genitourinary system diseases	(−)
Component 4			
Circulatory system diseases	(−)		
35 to 49 years	(−)		
Digestive system diseases	(+)		
50 to 64 years	(+)		
Respiratory system diseases	(+)		

(+) = positive correlation

(−) = negative correlation

personnel report of each hospital was used as the index of nursing education output; see appendix 1B for further details. The number of house staff in the hospital, as reported by the American Medical Association, was taken as the index of physician education output.[26] As with ambulatory visits, further disaggregation of the educational output measures was deemed undesirable.

These output levels of ambulatory patient care, nurse education, and physician education were converted into product-mix measures simply by dividing them by the level of inpatient care output. This yielded ten product-mix measures: the seven case-mix components (COMP1, . . . , COMP7), the number of ambulatory visits per case (AMB), the number of medical students per case (MEDUC), and the number of nursing students per case (NEDUC). These ten variables correspond to the p_j's discussed in the first section of this chapter.

This method of measuring product mix differs from the methods of the numerous studies of hospital costs that have used data on facilities and services offered by hospitals to adjust for interhospital differences in product mix.[27] Given the substantial case-mix information available for this study, it is doubtful that using the available facilities and services data in addition to the case-mix data would yield results sufficiently different to justify the additional costs involved. Also available data on facilities and services are minimal.[28]

A Crude Test of the Product-Mix Adjustment

It is impossible to assess the degree of correspondence between the ten product-mix measures and a complete representation of the output mix for each hospital; the data needed for such a complete representation do not exist. A less accurate but feasible method of testing the accuracy of these product-mix measures is to regress cost per case on them. If the product-mix measures explain a substantial amount of the interhospital variation in average cost per case, we may (at least tentatively) conclude that they are a fairly accurate representation of the complete product mix of each hospital.

Equations 1.3, 1.5, and 1.7 in table 1–5, estimated by ordinary least squares (OLS), indicate that product-mix measures explain 65 percent of the variation in average total cost per case (ATC), 61 percent of the variation in average labor cost per case (ALC), and 62 percent of the variation in average nonlabor cost per case (ANLC).[29] The associated F values are all significant at the 1 percent level.

The seven case-mix components account for 82 percent of the variation in the original case-mix variables. Further evidence that the components are a reasonably adequate representation of the original case-mix variables is presented in equations 1.4, 1.6, and 1.8 of table 1–5. The use of the original case-mix variables only explains an additional 10 percent, 16 percent, and 10 percent of the variations in ALC, ANLC, and ATC respectively.[30] Given the substantial loss in degrees of freedom that results from including all the original case-mix variables, the use of the principal components in their stead seems amply justified.

The Estimated Cost Functions

We now turn to the problem of estimating cross-sectional cost functions. After considering the functional forms employed, I shall present and discuss the results of estimating several alternative specifications by various estimation methods.

Table 1-5
1964 Average Cost per Case Regressed on Product-Mix Variables
(t-values in parentheses)

(1.3) ATC = 250.3 + 1.849 COMP 1 − 3.713 COMP 2 + 2.689 COMP 3 − 1.259 COMP 4 + 0.2793 COMP 5
       (4.89)   (3.06)   (4.50)   (2.51)   (0.99)   (0.22)
       + 2.207 COMP 6 + 4.428 COMP 7 + 13.58 AMB + 33,730 MEDUC − 2,174 NEDUC
       (1.52)   (2.45)   (3.05)   (4.55)   (0.92)

$R^2 = 0.65$
$F = 12.11$

(1.4) ATC = 499.6 + 1.889 CASE 1 − 2.168 CASE 2 − 8.744 CASE 3 + 2.502 CASE 4 + 1.419 CASE 5
       (0.85)   (1.32)   (0.88)   (1.77)   (1.00)   (0.62)
       + 1.375 CASE 6 − 1.324 CASE 7 − 8.096 CASE 8 − 0.7453 CASE 9 + 3.605 CASE 10
       (0.60)   (0.34)   (0.88)   (0.12)   (0.47)
       + 4.996 CASE 11 − 18.82 CASE 12 + 2.306 CASE 13 − 0.0873 CASE 14 − 2.142 CASE 15
       (0.69)   (1.32)   (0.24)   (0.01)   (0.36)
       − 7.171 CASE 16 − 1.846 CASE 17 − 6.721 CASE 18 − 5.643 CASE 19 − 9.999 CASE 20
       (1.19)   (0.31)   (1.07)   (0.81)   (0.95)
       − 3.664 CASE 21 − 8.731 CASE 22 + 11.40 CASE 23 + 2.074 CASE 24 − 3.301 CASE 25
       (0.44)   (0.72)   (0.67)   (0.23)   (0.51)
       + 0.8343 CASE 26 + 14.19 AMB + 25,780 MEDUC − 3,560 NEDUC
       (0.08)   (2.69)   (2.92)   (1.33)

$R^2 = 0.75$
$F = 4.79$

(1.5) ANLC = 66.45 + 0.8360 COMP 1 − 1.184 COMP 2 + 0.8514 COMP 3 − 0.0066 COMP 4 + 0.4714 COMP 5
      (3.95)   (4.20)   (4.36)   (2.41)   (0.02)   (1.11)
      + 0.5098 COMP 6 + 1.138 COMP 7 + 3.616 AMB + 10,460 MEDUC − 937.3 NEDUC
      (1.07)   (1.91)   (2.47)   (4.29)   (1.20)

      $R^2 = 0.62$
      $F = 10.45$

(1.6) ANLC = 135.3 + 0.6232 CASE 1 − 0.2825 CASE 2 − 3.413 CASE 3 + 1.697 CASE 4 + 1.107 CASE 5
      (0.78)   (1.46)   (0.38)   (2.32)   (2.28)   (1.64)
      + 1.634 CASE 6 − 0.7520 CASE 7 − 2.892 CASE 8 − 0.4692 CASE 9 − 0.3858 CASE 10
      (2.41)   (0.66)   (1.06)   (0.26)   (0.17)
      − 0.0504 CASE 11 − 7.94 CASE 12 + 0.726 CASE 13 − 0.2953 CASE 14 − 0.6035 CASE 15
      (0.02)   (1.87)   (0.25)   (0.15)   (0.34)
      − 3.099 CASE 16 − 1.436 CASE 17 − 1.197 CASE 18 − 2.789 CASE 19 − 3.685 CASE 20
      (1.73)   (0.80)   (0.64)   (1.34)   (1.18)
      − 0.8801 CASE 21 − 2.524 CASE 22 − 3.265 CASE 23 + 4.010 CASE 24 − 0.6327 CASE 25
      (0.36)   (0.70)   (0.65)   (1.50)   (0.33)
      + 1.177 CASE 26 + 2.955 AMB + 8,840 MEDUC − 1,383 NEDUC
      (0.38)   (1.88)   (3.36)   (1.73)

      $R^2 = 0.78$
      $F = 5.49$

(1.7) ALC = 183.9 + 1.013 COMP 1 − 2.531 COMP 2 + 1.839 COMP 3 − 1.254 COMP 4 + 0.1922 COMP 5
      (4.72) (2.20)   (4.03)   (2.25)   (1.29)   (0.20)
      + 1.699 COMP 6 + 3.292 COMP 7 + 9.965 AMB + 23,287 MEDUC − 1,237 NEDUC
      (1.54)   (2.39)   (2.93)   (4.12)   (0.68)

      $R^2 = 0.61$
      $F = 10.35$

Table 1–5 continued

$$
\begin{aligned}
\text{(1.8)} \quad \text{ALC} = 364.4 &+ 1.266 \text{ CASE 1} - 1.886 \text{ CASE 2} - 5.333 \text{ CASE 3} + 0.8054 \text{ CASE 4} + 0.3119 \text{ CASE 5} \\
&\;(0.80)\quad(1.13)\qquad\;\;(0.98)\qquad\;\;(1.38)\qquad\;\;(0.41)\qquad\quad(0.17) \\[4pt]
&- 0.2592 \text{ CASE 6} - 0.5726 \text{ CASE 7} - 5.207 \text{ CASE 8} - 0.2763 \text{ CASE 9} + 3.993 \text{ CASE 10} \\
&\quad(0.15)\qquad\quad(0.19)\qquad\;\;(0.72)\qquad\;\;(0.06)\qquad\;\;(0.67) \\[4pt]
&+ 5.049 \text{ CASE 11} - 10.89 \text{ CASE 12} + 1.581 \text{ CASE 13} + 0.3828 \text{ CASE 14} - 1.540 \text{ CASE 15} \\
&\quad(0.89)\qquad\quad(0.97)\qquad\;\;(0.21)\qquad\;\;(0.07)\qquad\;\;(0.33) \\[4pt]
&- 4.075 \text{ CASE 16} - 0.4111 \text{ CASE 17} - 5.527 \text{ CASE 18} - 2.854 \text{ CASE 19} - 6.317 \text{ CASE 20} \\
&\quad(0.86)\qquad\quad(0.09)\qquad\;\;(1.12)\qquad\;\;(0.52)\qquad\;\;(0.77) \\[4pt]
&- 2.785 \text{ CASE 21} - 6.210 \text{ CASE 22} + 14.68 \text{ CASE 23} - 1.937 \text{ CASE 24} - 2.670 \text{ CASE 25} \\
&\quad(0.43)\qquad\quad(0.65)\qquad\;\;(1.11)\qquad\;\;(0.27)\qquad\;\;(0.53) \\[4pt]
&- 0.3427 \text{ CASE 26} + 11.24 \text{ AMB} + 16{,}951 \text{ MEDUC} - 2{,}179 \text{ NEDUC} \\
&\quad(0.04)\qquad\qquad(2.72)\qquad\;\;(2.45)\qquad\qquad(1.04)
\end{aligned}
$$

$R^2 = 0.71$

$F = 3.87$

The Basic Functional Forms

The estimation process began by employing the following two functional forms

$$ATC = a_0 + a_1 BEDS + a_2(BEDS)^2 + a_3 FLOW + a_4(FLOW)^2$$
$$+ a_5 COMP1 + \ldots + a_{11} COMP7 + a_{12} AMB \qquad (1.9)$$
$$+ a_{13} MEDUC + a_{14} NEDUC + u$$

$$ATC = b_0 + b_1 BEDS + b_2(BEDS)^2 + b_3 Log(FLOW)$$
$$+ b_4 COMP1 + \ldots + b_{10} COMP7 + b_{11} AMB \qquad (1.10)$$
$$+ b_{12} MEDUC + b_{13} NEDUC + v$$

where the a's and b's are coefficients to be estimated, u and v are error terms, BEDS is the bed complement of each hospital, and FLOW is the case-flow rate of each hospital, that is, the number of inpatient cases divided by the number of beds. FLOW corresponds to U (the measure of capacity utilization), and BEDS corresponds to S (the measure of size).

The total cost function corresponding to equation 1.9 is

$$TC = \lambda'\delta + a_1 BEDS \cdot Q + a_2(BEDS)^2 \cdot Q$$
$$+ a_3 FLOW \cdot Q + a_4(FLOW)^2 \cdot Q \qquad (1.11)$$
$$+ a_{12} AMBVIS + a_{13} HSTAFF + a_{14} SNURSE + uQ$$

where AMBVIS is the total number of ambulatory visits, HSTAFF is the number of interns and residents in training programs, SNURSE is the number of student nurses, λ is a twenty-nine-element vector of case-type coefficients, δ is a twenty-nine-element vector of the number of cases in each case type, and Q is the total number of inpatient cases (lowercase Greek letters indicate vectors). Thus a_{12}, a_{13}, and a_{14} may be interpreted as the marginal costs of providing an additional outpatient visit, an additional year of physician training, and an additional year of nurse training respectively.

When BEDS is set equal to some number K, the marginal cost of treating a case of type i, j, k is $\lambda_i + \lambda_j + \lambda_k + a_1 K + a_2 K^2 + 2a_3 Y/K + 3a_4 Y^2/K^2$, where Y is a given level of Q and where λ_r is the rth element of λ.[31] Letting the rth element of π, which is also a twenty-nine-element column vector, be equal to $\lambda_r - \lambda_i - \lambda_j - \lambda_k$, we see that $\lambda'\delta = \pi'\delta + (\lambda_i + \lambda_j + \lambda_k) \cdot 3Q$. Using this equality to substitute for $\lambda'\delta$ and dividing both sides of equation 1.11 by Q yields

$$ATC = \pi'\gamma + 3(\lambda_i + \lambda_j + \lambda_k) + a_1 BEDS$$
$$+ a_2(BEDS)^2 + a_3 FLOW + a_4(FLOW)^2 + \qquad (1.12)$$
$$a_{12} AMB + a_{13} MEDUC + a_{14} NEDUC + u$$

where λ is a twenty-nine-element column vector of case-mix proportions.

Since three elements of γ, one each corresponding to an age category, a sex category, and a diagnostic category, are simply equal to one minus the other elements of γ that refer to the same kind of category, they may be eliminated from equation 1.12 by substituting for them and recomputing the coefficients of the remaining twenty-six case-mix proportions. Finally, to arrive at equation 1.9 we substitute for the remaining case-mix proportions the seven principal components described in table 1–2. This substitution requires that the recomputed coefficients of the remaining twenty-six case-mix proportions satisfy a set of nineteen linear relationships. Of course, in estimating the equations reported in the following sections, we have imposed the assumption that these relationships are in fact satisfied. Also equation 1.10 may be derived from a total cost function in an analogous manner.

The estimated average cost functions use ALC and ANLC as the dependent variables rather than ATC.[32] This procedure was necessary because the price of labor clearly differed across hospitals in the sample (both rural hospitals and New York City hospitals are included in the sample). To allow for this, wage indexes were computed for a number of geographic areas, and the reported labor costs of each hospital were adjusted by means of these indexes. The calculation of these indexes is described in appendix 1B. Specifically, the labor costs of non–New York City hospitals were multiplied by the ratio of the New York City index to the index for the geographic area in which each of these hospitals was located.[33] Of course, in calculating the effect of product-mix changes on inflation, the estimated ALC used in computing $\overline{AC}_{i64}$, was multiplied by the ratio of each hospital's index to the New York City index.[34]

It was also assumed that nonlabor input prices did not vary enough across the sample hospitals to warrant adjustment of reported nonlabor costs. This assumption is partly one of convenience. That is, there appears to be no straightforward way to correct for such differences in the absence of any information about the quantities of nonlabor inputs.

Results of the Cost Function Estimation

The results of estimating cost functions of the form shown in equations 1.9 and 1.10 are presented in table 1–6. The overall level of explanation of these equations is quite high. And they all display one surprising result, namely, that the effect of scale is to increase average cost until a size of approximately 300 beds is reached and to decrease average cost very slightly thereafter.

More specifically, the maximum-cost value for BEDS is 294.2, which is obtained by summing equations 1.13 and 1.15, differentiating with respect to BEDS, setting the result equal to zero, and solving for BEDS. By substituting sample means for all the independent variables except BEDS and $BEDS^2$ and by substituting 294.2 for BEDS and $(294.2)^2$ for $BEDS^2$, we obtain an average total cost per case of \$398.34. When BEDS is increased to the sample maximum of 452, this average cost decreases by \$24.90; and when BEDS is decreased from 294.2 to the sample minimum of 25, the decrease in average cost is \$72.47.[35]

While this pattern of scale effects has been found before, most studies of hospital costs have found either continuously negative scale effects or first negative and then positive scale effects on average cost.[36] The negative scale effects are usually attributed to production function characteristics (increasing returns to scale) while the positive scale effects are usually explained by management problems that occur in very large enterprises or institutions.[37]

The results in table 1–6 are difficult to explain in terms of production function characteristics or managerial problems in large enterprises. For example, we might assume that the average cost effect of managerial problems is largest in moving from very small hospitals to slightly larger ones and smallest in moving from very large hospitals to even larger ones. With continuously increasing returns to scale, this assumption would imply the pattern of scale effects shown in table 1–6. And while this assumption seems unreasonable, the only other interpretation of these results (in terms of scale effects and managerial-problems effects) is that the managerial-problems effect remains constant or increases with size while returns to scale increase more and more rapidly with size, or that returns to scale do in fact decrease and then increase. Neither interpretation is consistent with all the evidence cited from other studies.

A more reasonable interpretation of these results is that the attempt to adjust for product-mix differences was not completely successful. It may be that the diagnostic categories listed in table 1–1 are too broad and that, for example, patients treated for respiratory diseases in larger hospitals are on average more seriously ill than patients treated for respiratory disease in smaller hospitals. Alternatively, it may be that larger hospitals provide higher-quality treatment for exactly the same cases and therefore incur higher costs per case. In either case, failure to adjust for these output differences could easily explain the findings regarding scale effects.[38]

In summary, the coefficients of BEDS and $BEDS^2$ in table 1–6 should

Table 1–6
Estimated Cross-Sectional Cost Functions, 1964
(t-values in parentheses)

(1.13) ALC = 455.6 + 0.4671 BEDS − 0.0008 BEDS^2 − 12.45 FLOW + 0.1179 FLOW^2 − 1.174 COMP 2
         (7.58)   (2.37)   (1.84)   (4.19)   (3.03)   (2.02)

         + 1.084 COMP 3 − 0.6207 COMP 4 + 0.8711 COMP 6 + 1.094 COMP 7 + 5.279 AMB
           (1.42)   (0.74)   (0.90)   (0.93)   (1.60)

         + 15,165 MEDUC − 409.3 NEDUC
           (2.39)   (0.25)

R^2 = 0.74
F = 14.98

(1.14) ALC = 657.3 + 0.4654 BEDS − 0.0008 BEDS^2 − 139.5 Log(FLOW) − 0.9759 COMP 2 + 1.212 COMP 3
         (8.64)   (2.37)   (1.84)   (5.23)   (1.70)   (1.62)

         − 0.9053 COMP 4 + 0.6898 COMP 6 + 1.159 COMP 7 + 4.53 AMB + 15,860 MEDUC
           (1.11)   (0.72)   (0.99)   (1.40)   (2.53)

         − 804 NEDUC
           (0.49)

R^2 = 0.74
F = 16.51

(1.15) $ANLC = 134.4 + 0.1213\ BEDS - 0.0002\ BEDS^2 - 2.934\ FLOW + 0.0225\ FLOW^2 + 0.5043\ COMP\ 1$
  (4.189)   (1.334)   (0.98)   (2.06)   (1.26)   (2.25)

$- 0.668\ COMP\ 2 + 0.6558\ COMP\ 3 + 0.5602\ COMP\ 5 + 0.4649\ COMP\ 7 + 0.9871\ AMB$
  (2.46)   (1.87)   (1.49)   (0.84)   (0.65)

$+ 9{,}949\ MEDUC - 836.3\ NEDUC$
  (3.29)   (1.11)

$R^2 = 0.70$
$F = 12.50$

(1.16) $ANLC = 216.3 + 0.1217\ BEDS - 0.0002\ BEDS^2 - 44.03\ Log(FLOW) + 0.4984\ COMP\ 1 - 0.647\ COMP\ 2$
  (4.79)   (1.35)   (0.99)   (3.60)   (2.24)   (2.40)

$+ 0.6575\ COMP\ 3 + 0.5437\ COMP\ 5 + 0.4743\ COMP\ 7 + 0.9458\ AMB + 10{,}050\ MEDUC$
  (1.91)   (1.45)   (0.87)   (0.63)   (3.37)

$- 886.7\ NEDUC$
  (1.21)

$R^2 = 0.70$
$F = 13.86$

Note: These equations were estimated by ordinary least squares.

be interpreted as measuring the effect on cost of both changes in scale and the product-mix differences, not accounted for by product-mix variables, which are associated with size. Since we wish to use the estimated cost functions to adjust for product-mix change but not for scale change, it would be nice to be able to distinguish scale effects from unmeasured product-mix effects. Tables 1–7 and 1–8 report the results of attempts to include additional variables derived from BEDS in the hope that some of these variables would pick up scale effects while the others would measure omitted product-mix differences. As would be expected, collinearity among the variables defined from BEDS frustrated these efforts.[39]

In the light of the substantial evidence regarding the smallness of scale effects,[40] and in view of the fact that scale effects could not be successfully distinguished from unmeasured product-mix effects, it seems reasonable to interpret the coefficients of BEDS and BEDS^2 as representing primarily the latter type of effect.[41] But the inverted-U pattern suggests that unmeasured product-mix differences tend to decrease costs beyond a certain size level. Given that the unmeasured product-mix differences probably reflect differences in quality (however defined) or in severity of cases treated, this implication seems unreasonable.

Furthermore, the evidence for this negative effect on costs in the sample is rather weak. The magnitude of the decrease from 294.2 beds to the maximum bed size of 452 beds is relatively small. Also the estimated coefficients of BEDS^2 in table 1–6 do not always exceed their standard errors. On the other hand, if BEDS^2 were simply dropped from the estimated cost function, a linear pattern of cost increases due to unmeasured product-mix differences would be implied. It seems more reasonable to assume that the unmeasured product-mix differences diminish as size increases. That is, we expect the unmeasured product-mix differences between a 50-bed hospital and a 150-bed hospital to have a greater impact on average cost than the corresponding differences between a 350-bed hospital and a 450-bed hospital.[42]

To allow for a diminishing effect of unmeasured product-mix differences on cost as size increased, BEDS and BEDS^2 were replaced by BEDS^{-1} in the estimated cost functions. The results of this replacement are shown in equations 1.25 and 1.27 of table 1–9. Table 1–10 indicates that the relationship between predicted average cost and size (with other independent variables taking on their mean values) derived from these equations is quite similar to the pattern derived from equations 1.13 and 1.15. This table shows the relationship between predicted cost at various bed sizes and predicted cost at 294.2 beds (with other independent variables again set equal to their mean values). Finally notice that the values of R^2 in equations 1.25 and 1.27 of table 1–9 are almost identical to the values for equations 1.13 and 1.15.

These observations indicate that $BEDS^{-1}$ is an adequate substitute for BEDS and $BEDS^2$ and that it is preferable to BEDS and $BEDS^2$ on a priori grounds.[43]

Equations 1.26 and 1.28 enable us to test the significance of the product-mix variables (in addition to $BEDS^{-1}$) that are included in equations 1.25 and 1.27. For equations 1.25 and 1.26 the relevant F-value is 4.31, while for equations 1.27 and 1.28 it is 4.02. Both are significant at the 99 percent level.

However, several case-mix components have been dropped from these equations and from the others presented in this section. These components were dropped because their coefficients had extremely low t-values. But to preserve a reasonably complete description of each hospital's product mix, I arbitrarily adopted the rule that at least five components should be included in each equation. Thus the coefficients of some of the retained components do not exceed their standard errors in absolute value, yet they were not dropped from the relevant equations. Similarly, some of the coefficients of NEDUC and AMB do not exceed their standard errors in absolute value, but the variables were not dropped from the relevant equations in order to maintain accuracy in the representation of product mix. Equations 1.29 and 1.30 of table 1–11 indicate that when the product-mix variables with t-values less than one are dropped from equations 1.25 and 1.27, the coefficients of the other variables and the level of explanation (as measured by R^2) are virtually unaffected.

Most of the analysis that follows focuses on results obtained from cost functions using the specifications of equations 1.25 and 1.27. I used FLOW and $FLOW^2$ rather than Log(FLOW) because of the apparent absence of scale effects. In other words, for a given level of admission equations 1.31 and 1.32 indicate that the optimal bed size is zero because changes in scale affect only changes in average cost through changes in Log(FLOW).[44] If, on the other hand, the coefficient of Log(FLOW) were positive, the optimal bed size would be infinite. In equations 1.25 and 1.27, however, we may calculate the case-flow rate that minimizes average cost. By dividing the given number of admissions into this rate, we may determine the optimal bed size given this number of admissions.

By adding equations 1.25 and 1.27, differentiating with respect to FLOW, and setting the result equal to zero, we find that the case-flow rate that minimizes average cost is 59.2.[45] Not only is this optimal rate very high, it is also very close to (and not significantly different from) the maximum observed rate of 61.4.[46] In other words, the implication of the specification with Log(FLOW), that the impact of FLOW is negative over the range of observed values, is consistent with the results obtained when FLOW and $FLOW^2$ are used.

In conclusion, if the estimated cost functions are presumed to indicate

Table 1-7
1964 Cross-Sectional Cost Functions with BEDS, BEDS², and BEDS⁻¹

(1.17) ALC = 468.2 − 12.363 FLOW + 0.1168 FLOW² + 0.4003 BEDS − 0.0007 BEDS² − 416.9 BEDS⁻¹
              (6.06) (4.11)   (2.97)   (1.28)   (1.22)   (0.28)
            − 1.17 COMP 2 + 0.9786 COMP 3 − 0.6235 COMP 4 + 0.8817 COMP 6 + 1.21 COMP 7
              (2.00)   (1.14)   (0.74)   (0.90)   (0.96)
            + 5.2571 AMB + 15,382 MEDUC − 439.42 NEDUC
              (1.59)   (2.39)   (0.26)

$R^2 = 0.74$

(1.18) ANLC = 146.0 − 2.9335 FLOW + 0.0223 FLOW² + 0.0721 BEDS − 0.0001 BEDS² − 312.49 BEDS⁻¹
               (3.47) (2.05)   (1.24)   (0.49)   (0.46)   (0.43)
             + 0.4773 COMP 1 − 0.6592 COMP 2 + 0.5804 COMP 3 + 0.5559 COMP 5 + 0.5401 COMP 7
               (2.04)   (2.40)   (1.47)   (1.46)   (0.93)
             + 0.9676 AMB + 10,038 MEDUC − 850.31 NEDUC
               (0.63)   (3.29)   (1.12)

$R^2 = 0.71$

(1.19) ALC = 673.7 − 138.79 Log(FLOW) + 0.3788 BEDS − 0.0007 BEDS² − 541.95 BEDS⁻¹
              (7.53) (6.09)   (1.22)   (1.17)   (0.36)
            + 1.072 COMP 3 − 0.9036 COMP 4 + 0.7072 COMP 6 + 1.3088 COMP 7 − 0.9741 COMP 2
              (1.27)   (1.10)   (0.735)   (1.05)   (1.68)
            + 16,125 MEDUC − 837.10 NEDUC + 4.5159 AMB
              (2.54)   (0.51)   (1.38)

$R^2 = 0.74$

$$
\begin{aligned}
(1.20)\quad \text{ANLC} = 229.7 &- 44.535\ \text{Log(FLOW)} + 0.0717\ \text{BEDS} - 0.0001\ \text{BEDS}^2 - 319.02\ \text{BEDS}^{-1} + 0.4704\ \text{COMP 1} \\
&\quad (4.21)\qquad\qquad (3.66)\qquad\quad (0.50)\qquad\quad (0.46)\qquad\quad (0.44)\qquad\qquad (2.02) \\[4pt]
&- 0.6386\ \text{COMP 2} + 0.5792\ \text{COMP 3} + 0.5390\ \text{COMP 5} + 0.5512\ \text{COMP 7} + 0.9296\ \text{AMB} \\
&\quad (2.35)\qquad\qquad (1.49)\qquad\qquad (1.43)\qquad\qquad (0.96)\qquad\qquad (0.615) \\[4pt]
&+ 10{,}136\ \text{MEDUC} - 897.55\ \text{NEDUC} \\
&\quad (3.37)\qquad\qquad (1.21) \\[6pt]
&R^2 = 0.71
\end{aligned}
$$

Table 1–8
1964 Cross-Sectional Cost Functions with BEDS, Log(BEDS), and BEDS^{-1}
(t-vaues in parentheses)

(1.21) $ALC = 253.2 - 12.197\ FLOW + 0.1152\ FLOW^2 - 0.1775\ BEDS + 54.780\ Log(BEDS)$
       (0.76)   (3.05)   (0.04)   (0.30)   (0.76)
       $+ 764.90\ BEDS^{-1} - 1.1952\ COMP\ 2 + 0.9577\ COMP\ 3 - 0.6159\ COMP\ 4$
       (0.33)   (0.59)   (0.86)   (0.86)
       $+ 0.8515\ COMP\ 6 + 1.3128\ COMP\ 7 + 5.5187\ AMB + 15{,}428\ MEDUC$
       (0.98)   (1.28)   (3.35)   (6,480)
       $- 597.12\ NEDUC$
       (1,674)

        $R^2 = 0.74$

(1.22) $ANLC = 68.90 - 2.9793\ FLOW + 0.0228\ FLOW^2 - 0.0643\ BEDS + 18.511\ Log(BEDS)$
        (0.44)   (2.07)   (1.26)   (0.47)   (0.55)
       $+ 280.61\ BEDS^{-1} + 0.4815\ COMP\ 1 - 0.6536\ COMP\ 2 + 0.5786\ COMP\ 3$
       (0.18)   (2.06)   (2.38)   (1.47)
       $+ 0.5296\ COMP\ 5 + 0.5260\ COMP\ 7 + 0.9250\ AMB + 10{,}072\ MEDUC$
       (1.38)   (0.90)   (0.60)   (3.30)
       $- 854.95\ NEDUC$
       (1.13)

        $R^2 = 0.71$

(1.23) $ALC = 468.5 - 137.19 \ Log(FLOW) - 0.1694 \ BEDS + 51.827 \ Log(BEDS) + 570.98 \ BEDS^{-1}$
        (1.45)   (5.90)   (0.57)   (0.72)   (0.17)

$- 1.0003 \ COMP \ 2 + 1.0505 \ COMP \ 3 - 0.8914 \ COMP \ 4 + 0.6800 \ COMP \ 6$
  (1.71)   (1.23)   (1.08)   (0.70)

$+ 1.4045 \ COMP \ 7 + 4.7770 \ AMB + 16,147 \ MEDUC - 982.29 \ NEDUC$
  (1.11)   (1.45)   (2.53)   (0.60)

$R^2 = 0.74$

(1.24) $ANLC = 150.4 - 44.972 \ Log(FLOW) - 0.0660 \ BEDS + 19.067 \ Log(BEDS) + 300.67 \ BEDS^{-1}$
        (0.97)   (3.619)   (0.49)   (0.58)   (0.19)

$+ 0.4748 \ COMP \ 1 - 0.6308 \ COMP \ 2 + 0.5784 \ COMP \ 3 + 0.5116 \ COMP \ 5$
  (2.04)   (2.31)   (1.49)   (1.35)

$+ 0.5770 \ COMP \ 7 + 0.8754 \ AMB + 10,174 \ MEDUC - 903.07 \ NEDUC$
  (0.92)   (0.58)   (3.38)   (1.23)

$R^2 = 0.71$

Table 1–9
1964 Cross-Sectional Cost Functions with FLOW, FLOW², and BEDS⁻¹
(t-values in parentheses)

(1.25) $\text{ALC} = 505.4 - 11.536 \text{ FLOW} + 0.1087 \text{ FLOW}^2 - 1910.7 \text{ BEDS}^{-1} - 1.2787 \text{ COMP 2}$
$\qquad\qquad (7.16) \quad\; (3.95) \qquad\qquad (2.82) \qquad\qquad (2.27) \qquad\qquad (221)$
$\qquad\qquad\qquad\qquad\qquad + 0.8647 \text{ COMP 3} - 0.5904 \text{ COMP 4} + 0.8513 \text{ COMP 6} + 1.6611 \text{ COMP 7}$
$\qquad\qquad\qquad\qquad\qquad\; (1.05) \qquad\qquad (0.70) \qquad\qquad (0.87) \qquad\qquad (1.40)$
$\qquad\qquad\qquad\qquad\qquad + 5.8875 \text{ AMB} + 16{,}551 \text{ MEDUC} - 604.99 \text{ NEDUC}$
$\qquad\qquad\qquad\qquad\qquad\; (1.82) \qquad\quad (2.83) \qquad\qquad (0.38)$

$\qquad\qquad R^2 = 0.73$

(1.26) $\text{ALC} = 647.8 - 14.673 \text{ FLOW} + 0.1248 \text{ FLOW}^2 - 4247.2 \text{ BEDS}^{-1}$
$\qquad\qquad (10.97) \quad (4.69) \qquad\qquad (2.98) \qquad\qquad (6.30)$

$\qquad\qquad R^2 = 0.59$

(1.27) $\text{ANLC} = 154.5 - 2.8221 \text{ FLOW} + 0.0211 \text{ FLOW}^2 - 594.39 \text{ BEDS}^{-1} + 0.4583 \text{ COMP 1}$
$\qquad\qquad\; (4.21) \quad\; (2.02) \qquad\qquad (1.20) \qquad\qquad (1.53) \qquad\qquad (2.05)$
$\qquad\qquad\qquad\qquad\qquad - 0.6742 \text{ COMP 2} + 0.5562 \text{ COMP 3} + 0.5543 \text{ COMP 5} + 0.6191 \text{ COMP 7}$
$\qquad\qquad\qquad\qquad\qquad\; (2.51) \qquad\qquad (1.48) \qquad\qquad (1.49) \qquad\qquad (1.13)$
$\qquad\qquad\qquad\qquad\qquad + 1.0713 \text{ AMB} + 10.222 \text{ MEDUC} - 871.36 \text{ NEDUC}$
$\qquad\qquad\qquad\qquad\qquad\; (0.73) \qquad\quad (3.64) \qquad\qquad (1.22)$

$\qquad\qquad R^2 = 0.70$

(1.28) $\text{ANLC} = 270.2 - 5.3777 \text{ FLOW} + 0.0404 \text{ FLOW}^2 - 1696.5 \text{ BEDS}^{-1}$
$\qquad\qquad\; (10.14) \quad (3.81) \qquad\qquad (2.14) \qquad\qquad (5.58)$

$\qquad\qquad R^2 = 0.56$

Table 1–10
Comparison of Patterns of Unmeasured Product-Mix Effects

Bed Size	Equations 1.13 and 1.15	Equations 1.25 and 1.27
25	−18.2	−23.8
50	−15.0	−10.8
75	−12.1	− 6.5
100	− 9.5	− 4.3
125	− 7.2	− 3.0
150	− 5.2	− 2.1
175	− 3.6	− 1.5
200	− 2.2	− 1.0
225	− 1.2	− 0.7
250	− 0.5	− 0.4
275	− 0.1	− 0.2
300	− 0.01	+ 0.04
325	− 0.2	+ 0.2
350	− 0.8	+ 0.4
375	− 1.6	+ 0.5
400	− 2.8	+ 0.6
425	− 4.3	+ 0.7
450	− 6.3	+ 0.8

Note: Percentage deviations from predicted cost at 294.2 beds.

only relationships within the observed ranges of variation for the independent variables, the use of Log(FLOW) cannot be rejected because it yields results almost identical to those obtained when FLOW and FLOW^2 are used. If these functions are presumed to indicate relationships both within and beyond the observed ranges of variation, then the absence of scale effects implies that the use of Log(FLOW) should be rejected on a priori grounds. But with the use of FLOW and FLOW^2 either interpretation of the cost functions may be retained.

Instrumental Variables and
Generalized Least-Squares Estimates

These equations were estimated by ordinary least squares (OLS). There is reason to believe that the coefficient estimates in these equations may be inconsistent because FLOW is an endogenous variable. For example, if hospital admissions are not completely price-inelastic and if prices are related to average costs, then a large positive error term for a particular hospital results in a low case-flow rate.[47]

An instrumental-variables approach was therefore used to obtain coefficient estimates more likely to be consistent than those obtained by

Table 1–11
Other 1964 Cross-Sectional Cost Functions Used for Adjusting Inflation Rates
(*t-values in parentheses*)

(1.29) $ALC = 504.2 - 12.269\ FLOW + 0.1162\ FLOW^2 - 1767.9\ BEDS^{-1} - 1.2439\ COMP\ 2$
$\qquad\qquad\ (7.60)\quad (4.52)\qquad\qquad (3.23)\qquad\qquad (2.17)\qquad\qquad (2.20)$
$\qquad\qquad\qquad + 0.9494\ COMP\ 3 + 1.4821\ COMP\ 7 + 5.9406\ AMB + 15,480\ MEDUC$
$\qquad\qquad\qquad\quad (1.17)\qquad\qquad (1.30)\qquad\qquad (1.89)\qquad\ (2.80)$

$\qquad\qquad R^2 = 0.73$

(1.30) $ANLC = 157.0 - 2.77\ FLOW + 0.0200\ FLOW^2 - 643.13\ BEDS^{-1} + 0.4566\ COMP\ 1$
$\qquad\qquad\qquad (4.31)\quad (1.99)\qquad\quad (1.15)\qquad\qquad (1.69)\qquad\qquad (2.05)$
$\qquad\qquad\qquad - 0.6058\ COMP\ 2 + 0.5460\ COMP\ 3 + 0.5150\ COMP\ 5 + 0.7163\ COMP\ 7$
$\qquad\qquad\qquad\quad (2.42)\qquad\qquad (1.46)\qquad\qquad (1.40)\qquad\qquad (1.36)$
$\qquad\qquad\qquad + 11,484\ MEDUC - 927.57\ NEDUC$
$\qquad\qquad\qquad\quad (5.23)\qquad\qquad (1.32)$

$\qquad\qquad R^2 = 0.70$

(1.31) $ALC = 698.5 - 130.87\ Log(FLOW) - 1946.9\ BEDS^{-1} - 1.0897\ COMP\ 2 + 0.9590\ COMP\ 3$
$\qquad\qquad\ (8.08)\quad (6.06)\qquad\qquad\quad (2.33)\qquad\qquad (1.92)\qquad\qquad (1.18)$
$\qquad\qquad\qquad - 0.8491\ COMP\ 4 + 0.6904\ COMP\ 6 + 1.7246\ COMP\ 7 + 5.1762\ AMB$
$\qquad\qquad\qquad\quad (1.04)\qquad\qquad (0.72)\qquad\qquad (1.47)\qquad\qquad (1.63)$
$\qquad\qquad\qquad + 17,130\ MEDUC - 973.46\ NEDUC$
$\qquad\qquad\qquad\quad (2.97)\qquad\qquad (0.63)$

$\qquad\qquad R^2 = 0.73$

(1.32) $ANLC = 237.3 - 43.584\ Log(FLOW) - 602.01\ BEDS^{-1} + 0.4505\ COMP\ 1 - 0.6553\ COMP\ 2$
$\qquad\qquad\qquad (4.68)\quad (3.62)\qquad\qquad\quad (1.56)\qquad\qquad (2.03)\qquad\qquad (2.46)$
$\qquad\qquad\qquad + 0.5525\ COMP\ 3 + 0.5370\ COMP\ 5 + 0.6286\ COMP\ 7 + 1.0379\ AMB$
$\qquad\qquad\qquad\quad (1.50)\qquad\qquad (1.46)\qquad\qquad (1.16)\qquad\qquad (0.71)$
$\qquad\qquad\qquad + 10,319\ MEDUC - 909.05\ NEDUC$
$\qquad\qquad\qquad\quad (3.73)\qquad\qquad (1.31)$

$\qquad\qquad R^2 = 0.70$

OLS. The first step of this procedure was to estimate OLS regressions in which FLOW and FLOW^2 were the dependent variables. The hospitals were ranked according to the value of FLOW and grouped into four groups and into ten groups with integers (1 to 4 and 1 to 10) assigned to each hospital depending on the groups in which it was included. These group numbers were used as independent variables in the Flow and FLOW^2 regressions. Other independent variables in these regressions were AMB, MNEDUC, NEDUC, BEDS^{-1}, and the seven case-mix components.

In the second step the predicted values of FLOW and FLOW^2 obtained from these OLS regressions were used as instruments in estimating equations identical to equations 1.25 and 1.27. The following results were obtained.

$$ALC = 326.9 - 2.341 \text{ FLOW} \quad - 0.0144 \text{ FLOW}^2 \quad - 1582.2 \text{ BEDS}^{-1}$$
$$(0.85) \quad (0.11) \qquad\qquad (0.04) \qquad\qquad (1.70)$$

$$+ 4.6873 \text{ AMB} \quad + 19{,}486 \text{ MEDUC} - 1462.5 \text{ NEDUC}$$
$$(0.90) \qquad\qquad (2.73) \qquad\qquad (0.58)$$

$$- 1.1909 \text{ COMP 2} + 1.2321 \text{ COMP 3} - 1.2929 \text{ COMP 4}$$
$$(1.24) \qquad\qquad (1.04) \qquad\qquad (0.71)$$

$$+ 0.6957 \text{ COMP 6} + 2.0424 \text{ COMP 7} \qquad\qquad (1.33)$$
$$(0.49) \qquad\qquad (1.52)$$

$R^2 = 0.69$

$$ANLC = 104.7 - 0.0409 \text{ FLOW} \quad - 0.0188 \text{ FLOW}^2 \quad - 578.29 \text{ BEDS}^{-1}$$
$$(1.19) \quad (0.01) \qquad\qquad (0.30) \qquad\qquad (1.39)$$

$$+ 0.6649 \text{ AMB} \quad + 10{,}772 \text{ MEDUC} - 1201.5 \text{ NEDUC}$$
$$(0.40) \qquad\qquad (3.41) \qquad\qquad (1.34)$$

$$+ 0.4928 \text{ COMP 1} - 0.5905 \text{ COMP 2} + 0.6526 \text{ COMP 3}$$
$$(1.92) \qquad\qquad (1.92) \qquad\qquad (1.56)$$

$$+ 0.5708 \text{ COMP 5} + 0.6789 \text{ COMP 7} \qquad\qquad (1.34)$$
$$(1.47) \qquad\qquad (1.16)$$

$R^2 = 0.68$

Two aspects of these results are worth noting here. First the coefficients of FLOW and FLOW^2 are very small relative to their standard errors, and the sign of the coefficient of FLOW^2 is different from that shown in table 1–9. Second, the coefficients of the product-mix variables (including BEDS^{-1}) are of the same sign and similar in magnitude to the corresponding coefficients in table 1–9. The sole exception is the coefficient of COMP 4 in the ALC equations. This implies that even if the OLS estimates are in fact inconsistent, replacing them by consistent estimates would make very little difference in the calculation of the impact of product-mix change on inflation.[48]

ALC ranged from \$148.21 to \$490.63 when adjusted for wage rate differences, while ANLC ranged from \$76.87 to \$219.74. Since the variations in both ALC and ANLC are large, there is reason to expect that the error terms in the average cost functions are heteroskedastic. This implies that the OLS estimates in equations 1.25 and 1.27 are inefficient. A test for the presence of heteroskedasticity was therefore performed.[49] The test statistics (10.15 for ALC and 7.93 for ANLC), distributed as chi-square with three degrees of freedom, were significantly different from zero at the 99 percent and 95 percent levels of significance for ALC and ANLC respectively, thus indicating the presence of substantial heteroskedasticity. Feldstein's method for obtaining efficient estimates was therefore employed. According to this method, observations are ranked according to predicted values of the dependent variable and then grouped (in this case into quartiles). Each observation is then weighted by the reciprocal of the maximum-likelihood estimate of the standard deviation in the error term for the group into which the observation falls. After dividing each observation by the mean of these weights (so that the average weight is equal to one), OLS is applied to the weighted observations.[50] In ascending order of predicted ALC, the quartile weights used here were 1.5436, 0.9063, 0.7346, and 0.8156. The corresponding weights for predicted ANLC were 1.2468, 1.0821, 0.6869, and 0.9841.

Applying OLS to the weighted observations yielded the following results.

$$ALC = 497.9 - 10.773 \text{ FLOW} + 0.0958 \text{ FLOW}^2 - 1950.8 \text{ BEDS}^{-1}$$
$$(7.48) \quad (4.00) \qquad\qquad (2.81) \qquad\qquad (2.72)$$

$$+ 5.6906 \text{ AMB} + 15,773 \text{ MEDUC} - 576.16 \text{ NEDUC}$$
$$(1.79) \qquad\qquad (2.70) \qquad\qquad (0.36)$$

$$- 1.0482 \text{ COMP 2} + 0.8131 \text{ COMP 3} - 0.7360 \text{ COMP 4}$$
$$(2.13) \qquad\qquad (1.05) \qquad\qquad (0.94)$$

$$+ 0.8784 \text{ COMP 6} + 1.0297 \text{ COMP 7} \qquad\qquad (1.35)$$
$$(1.02) \qquad\qquad (1.08)$$

$$R^2 = 0.76$$

$$ANLC = 153.5 - 2.944 \text{ FLOW} + 0.0225 \text{ FLOW}^2 - 542.78 \text{ BEDS}^{-1}$$
$$(4.44) \quad (2.28) \qquad\qquad (1.42) \qquad\qquad (1.53)$$

$$+ 0.8065 \text{ AMB} + 10,612 \text{ MEDUC} - 818.7 \text{ NEDUC}$$
$$(0.56) \qquad\qquad (3.95) \qquad\qquad (1.18)$$

$$+ \ 0.4383 \ \text{COMP} \ 1 \ - \ 0.5854 \ \text{COMP} \ 2 \ + \ 0.5899 \ \text{COMP} \ 3$$
$$(2.10) \qquad\qquad\quad (2.37) \qquad\qquad\quad (1.66)$$

$$+ \ 0.6245 \ \text{COMP} \ 5 \ + \ 0.5722 \ \text{COMP} \ 7 \qquad\qquad (1.36)$$
$$(1.80) \qquad\qquad\quad (1.12)$$

$R^2 = 0.74.$

After these equations were estimated, the test for heteroskedasticity was again performed. The test statistics, 4.968 for ALC and 0.887 for ANLC, were much lower than those for the original OLS estimates, although the hypothesis of homoskedasticity for the ALC equation could still be rejected at the 90 percent level of significance. The results shown in equations 1.14 and 1.15, however, are very similar to those in table 1–9. Since further attempts to eliminate heteroskedasticity in the ALC equation would clearly not alter these results in any important way, these attempts were not undertaken.

Further Remarks on the Estimated Cost Functions

In all the cost functions presented so far similar relationships between average cost per case and the product-mix variables were observed. That is, the estimated coefficients of the product-mix variables are stable in the sense that they do not change very much with changes in specification or method of estimation.

The coefficients of AMB, MEDUC, and NEDUC are of particular interest because they may be interpreted as marginal costs. Thus the marginal cost of an ambulatory patient visit seems to be approximately $6 or $7 while the cost of an additional year of nursing education is about $1,000.[51] Most striking, however, is that the estimate of the marginal cost of a year of physician's education is approximately $25,000. This figure is clearly larger than any direct expenditures associated with medical education programs. Why then do we observe such a high marginal cost for medical education?

One explanation is that in hospitals with teaching programs, the rate at which patients move through various stages of the treatment process depends on the requirements of the educational process. The result is that patients tend to have longer lengths of stay.[52] To test this explanation the following equation was estimated:

$$\text{LOS} = 21.95 \ - \ 0.5817 \ \text{FLOW} \ + \ 0.0060 \ \text{FLOW}^2 \ + \ 515.63 \ \text{MEDUC}$$
$$(10.51) \quad (7.22) \qquad\qquad (5.96) \qquad\qquad\quad (4.10)$$

$$+ \ 0.0446 \ \text{COMP} \ 1 \ - \ 0.0384 \ \text{COMP} \ 2 \ - \ 0.0332 \ \text{COMP} \ 3$$
$$(3.51) \qquad\qquad\quad (2.74) \qquad\qquad\quad (1.60)$$

$$- 0.0125 \text{ COMP } 4 + 0.0126 \text{ COMP } 5 + 0.0429 \text{ CCOMP } 6$$
$$(0.59) \qquad\qquad (0.62) \qquad\qquad (1.72)$$

$$+ 0.0429 \text{ COMP } 6 + 0.0322 \text{ COMP } 7 - 28.132 \text{ BEDS}^{-1}$$
$$(1.72) \qquad\qquad (1.09) \qquad\qquad (1.33)$$

$$R^2 = 0.84, \qquad\qquad\qquad\qquad\qquad\qquad\qquad\qquad\qquad (1.37)$$

where LOS is length of stay. The positive and highly significant coefficient for MEDUC suggests that this explanation is correct.

Since average cost per case (total cost/cases) is the product of average cost per day (total cost/days) and average length of stay (days/cases), a change of x percent in average length of stay will imply a change of x percent in average cost per case. Thus if the elasticity of LOS with respect to MEDUC is equal to the elasticity of ATC with respect to MEDUC, we may conclude that all the impact of MEDUC on ATC arises from its impact on LOS. By using equations 1.35, 1.36, and 1.37 and the facts that the sample means for MEDUC, ATC, and LOS are 0.00078, 375.93, and 8.49 respectively, we may calculate elasticities at the means for both LOS and ATC with respect to MEDUC.[53] These elasticities, 0.047 and 0.054 respectively, indicate that almost all the impact of MEDUC on ATC arises from its impact on LOS.

I have suggested that medical education programs cause patients to stay longer and that this longer stay explains the high marginal cost of a year of physician education. There are two reasons why this cost may actually be overstated. One is that the causal mechanism just postulated does not in fact exist and that the relationship between LOS and MEDUC arises from the fact that more serious cases are treated in hospitals with more extensive teaching programs. In other words, the case-mix data are too crude to pick up these differences in actual case mix, and since they are correlated with MEDUC, the estimated coefficients of MEDUC in the ALC and ANLC equations are biased upward. This objection could of course be tested against evidence gleaned from a thorough comparison of cases in various hospitals.

The second objection is somewhat more difficult to test. This is that higher-quality care (however defined) is given in hospitals with larger teaching programs. And the positive correlation between quality and MEDUC combined with the omission of measures of quality from the estimated cost functions biases the coefficients of MEDUC upward. To test this objection we would have to define and measure the quality of care in the sample hospitals.

Given the rapidly rising levels of hospital costs, the growth of medical education programs, and the national commitment to expanding these programs, a more extensive analysis of the costs of medical education is clearly needed. I have found some evidence that these costs may be larger than is usually reckoned because of the impact of medical education programs on the operations of the hospitals in which they are conducted. But further study of this question, and especially detailed study of specific hospitals with teaching programs, is clearly required. For a further analysis of the impact of medical education on average costs, see appendix 1A.

The Impact of Product-Mix Change on Rates of Cost Inflation

The estimated cost functions will now be used to calculate the impact of product-mix change on rates of cost inflation. The strategy is to use these functions to estimate the observed average cost in each hospital in 1964 if it had produced the same mix of products as it produced in 1961. This estimated cost is then divided by the observed average cost in 1961; then subtracting one from the result yields the rate of cost inflation for each hospital defined for its 1961 product mix. The results of these calculations are presented in table 1–12.

Explanation of Adjustment Methods

I argued in the preceding section that $BEDS^{-1}$ should be interpreted as a product-mix variable. This implies that $\overline{AC}_{i64}$ should be calculated on the assumption that $BEDS^{-1}$ takes on its 1961 observed value. But is this implication reasonable? Is it reasonable to argue that every time a hospital increases its bed complement by, say, five beds its product mix also changes even if the values of AMB, MEDUC, NEDUC, and the seven case-mix components are unchanged? Alternatively, we might argue that the unmeasured product-mix characteristics associated with size are long-run in nature. That is, product-mix changes associated with changes in size occur sometime after the actual expansion. When a fifty-bed hospital adds twenty-five beds it continues, for some time, to "act like" a fifty-bed hospital. Eventually, however, it acquires the capability to provide the services characteristic of a seventy-five-bed hospital.

   Except for cases of major capital expansion programs, which include the addition of more facilities and services as well as more beds, the lagged model of product-mix change seems plausible. If the lag is long enough, little of this adjustment will take place during the three-year period under consideration. Thus it seems preferable to calculate $\overline{AC}_{i64}$ on the assumption that $BEDS^{-1}$ takes on its 1964 value. This calculation

Table 1–12
Mean Adjusted Inflation Rates, 1961–1964
(in percent)

Adjustment Method		Inflation Rate
I	Unadjusted	27.77
II	Equations 1.25, 1.27, without Beds	25.35
III	Adjustment method II, with Beds	24.75
IV	Equations 1.31, 1.32, without Beds	25.46
V	Adjustment method IV, with Beds	24.85
VI	Equations 1.29, 1.30, without Beds	25.86
VII	Adjustment method VI, with Beds	25.28
VIII	Equations 1.17, 1.18, without Beds	25.61
IX	Adjustment method VIII, with Beds	24.69
X	Equations 1.21, 1.22, without Beds	25.70
XI	Adjustment method X, with Beds	25.52
XII	Instrumental variables, without Beds	25.40
XIII	Adjustment method XII, with Beds	24.88
XIV	GLS, without Beds	25.74
XV	GLS, with Beds	25.15
XVI	OLS, AMB only	27.00
XVII	OLS, MEDUC only	27.32
XVIII	OLS, NEDUC only	27.70
XIX	OLS, case-mix only	26.64
XX	OLS, beds only	27.17
XXI	GLS, AMB only	27.05
XXII	GLS, MEDUC only	27.32
XXIII	GLS, NEDUC only	27.71
XXIV	GLS, case-mix only	26.97
XXV	GLS, beds only	27.17

would exclude the effect of changes between 1961 and 1964 in BEDS^{-1} in keeping with the model of lagged product-mix change.

It is, of course, impossible to test empirically the lagged product-mix change hypothesis because it refers to characteristics of product mix that we have been unable to measure. Table 1–13 shows that a number of the hospitals in the sample experienced major capital expansions. While thirty-eight of the seventy-three hospitals remained in the same size class, fifteen others moved up at least two size classes from 1961 to 1964.[54]

In short, it seems impossible to determine whether it is correct to use the 1961 value for BEDS^{-1} (thus assuming that unmeasured product-mix characteristics changed within a hospital over the period and adjusting for these changes) or to use the 1964 value (thus assuming that these characteristics did not change). Table 1–12 therefore presents mean values for rates of cost inflation adjusted for product-mix change calculated in both ways. In the listing of adjustment methods in this table, the phrase

Table 1–13
Cross Tabulation of Sample Hospitals by Bed-Size Class, 1961 and 1964

1961 Bed-Size Class	1964 Bed-Size Class																	
	1	2	3	4	5	6	7	8	9	10	11	12	13	14	15	16	17	18
1	7	3																
2		6	2	2														
3			6	2														
4			1	1	1		1											
5					4	1												
6					1	2			1	1								
7							3	2	2		1							
8							3	3	2		1							
9								2	1									
10									1	2							1	
11									1	1	1							
12											2	1						
13																		
14																		
15																		
16																		1
17																		
18																		

Note: Bed-size class definitions: 1, 26–50; 2, 51–75; 3, 76–100; 4, 101–125; 5, 126–150; 6, 151–175; 7, 176–200; 8, 201–225; 9, 226–250; 10, 251–275; 11, 276–300; 12, 301–325; 13, 326–350; 14, 351–375; 15, 376–400; 16, 401–425; 17, 426–450; 18, 451+.

"without BEDS" indicates that the 1964 value for $BEDS^{-1}$ was used. The phrase "with BEDS" indicates that the 1961 value was used.

Notice also that in equations 1.21 and 1.22 the coefficient of $BEDS^{-1}$ was interpreted as representing scale effects while the coefficients of BEDS and Log(BEDS) were interpreted as representing the effects of unmeasured product-mix differences.[55] Thus adjustment method XI in table 1–12 uses the 1964 value for $BEDS^{-1}$ but the 1961 values for BEDS and Log(BEDS).

Adjustment methods XII and XIII use the coefficients of equations 1.33 and 1.34 while methods XIV and XV use the coefficients of equations 1.35 and 1.36. Methods XVI–XX use the coefficients of equations 1.25 and 1.27; methods XXI–XXV use equations 1.35 and 1.36. In methods XVI–XXV some of the product-mix variables are assumed to take on their 1964 values. For example, AMB, MEDUC, NEDUC, and $BEDS^{-1}$ in method XIX are assigned their 1964 values while the case-mix components take on their 1961 values. (The 1961 case-mix components were defined by the coefficients given in table 1–2.)

Results

The mean rate of inflation in observed average cost among the sample hospitals was 27.77 percent. The impact of the measured product-mix changes was to increase observed inflation rates by approximately 2 percent. According to adjustment method II in table 1–12, for example, the impact of measured product-mix change was 27.77 percent − 25.35 percent = 2.42 percent. The impact of unmeasured product-mix changes (as indicated by changes in $BEDS^{-1}$) was an additional increase of slightly over 0.5 percent. According to adjustment method III, for example, this impact was 25.35 percent − 24.75 percent = 0.60 percent.

The adjustment methods listed in table 1–12 indicate that the impact of product-mix change (both measured and unmeasured) was to increase observed rates of cost inflation by about 2.5 percent or 3 percent. Thus the mean rate of increase in the average cost of producing the composite product produced by each hospital in 1961 seems to be on the order of 25 percent. (These composite products differed across hospitals.) All the adjustment methods give roughly similar results. This is simply another reflection of the stability of the estimated coefficients for the product-mix variables.

At this point some comments about the interpretation of these results are in order. These results provide an answer to the following question: If all other relevant changes over the period 1961–1964 in fact took place, what would the observed rate of cost inflation have been if no product-mix change had occurred? The difference between this rate and the observed rate is the measure of the impact of product-mix change on inflation. It is also possible to ask, if none of the relevant changes over the 1961–1964 period in fact occurred, what would the observed rate of inflation have been if only product mix had changed? This rate might also be interpreted as the impact of product-mix change on inflation. Since this impact would presumably be measured by $(\overline{AC_{i61}/AC_{i61}}) - 1$, and since the impact of product-mix change was measured by $(AC_{i64}/AC_{i61}) - (\overline{AC_{i64}/AC_{i61}})$, we can readily see that our measure of this impact will be the larger one provided that $AC_{i64} - \overline{AC_{i64}}$ is greater than $\overline{AC_{i61}} - AC_{i61}$. In other words, the measure is larger if the absolute impact of product-mix change is larger according to the 1964 estimated cost function than according to a cost function estimated from 1961 data. Since this absolute impact is positive in 1964 and since increases in input prices over the 1961–1964 period suggest increasing marginal costs for outputs of various kinds, this condition is probably satisfied.

Adjustment methods XVI–XXV indicate that all types of product-mix change contributed to observed inflation. Increases in ambulatory visits per case accounted for an increase of about 0.75 percent. Increases in

MEDUC and decreases in NEDUC accounted for cost increases on the order of 0.45 percent and 0.06 percent respectively. Case-mix changes accounted for an increase of about 1.0 percent while changes in unmeasured product-mix characteristics (adjustment methods XX and XXV) accounted for an increase of about 0.6 percent.

While all types of product-mix changes were inflationary, their overall impact on observed inflation was not large. According to my calculations, about one-tenth of observed inflation can be attributed to the impact of product-mix change. But table 1–14 indicates that this result should not be surprising. The relative changes in almost all the mean values for product-mix variables used in this study were small. The primary exceptions are COMP 1, COMP 4, and COMP 7.[56]

In view of the hypotheses and conclusions of other students of hospital cost inflation, this conclusion does seem surprising. Thus it should be treated with caution. The emphasis on quality change in the hospital cost inflation literature seems to cast doubt on my results because I have not included a measure of quality and thus have not taken explicit account of quality change.[57] That is, since quality change is an aspect of product-mix change and since I have ignored this aspect, my results should understate the magnitude of the impact of product-mix change on inflation.

On the other hand, the unmeasured product-mix characteristics represented by $BEDS^{-1}$ in the estimated cost functions certainly include characteristics usually contained in the notion of quality. Thus this model does take account of quality differences that are correlated with size differences by including $BEDS^{-1}$. Any understatement in my results would therefore arise only from quality changes that are not associated with size changes. In other words, quality change between 1961 and 1964 may be divided into two types: (1) the changes that occurred when, for example, the typical 50-bed hospital of 1961 expanded to become, in 1964,

Table 1–14
Mean Product Mix, 1961 and 1964

	1961	1964
AMB	2.83	3.14
MEDUC	0.725×10^{-3}	0.782×10^{-3}
NEDUC	0.179×10^{-2}	0.166×10^{-2}
COMP 1	16.994	21.430
COMP 2	12.128	12.523
COMP 3	34.586	33.642
COMP 4	0.475	0.294
COMP 5	20.751	19.331
COMP 6	−15.549	−14.403
COMP 7	− 0.316	0.953

the typical 100-bed hospital of 1961; and (2) the changes that occurred when the typical 100-bed hospital of 1961 became the typical 100-bed hospital of 1964. By including BEDS^{-1} we can measure the impact of the first type of quality change on inflation. We cannot measure the impact of the second type of quality change.

Product-Mix Change and Reimbursement Methods

These results have some interesting implications for two notions regarding reimbursement methods that have appeared in the recent literature. One is the idea of grouping hospitals for purposes of computing reimbursement rates.[58] The other is Waldman's plan for reimbursing hospitals according to average increases in costs for the hospitals in the groups into which each hospital falls.[59] According to one variant of this plan, the reimbursable expense for the ith hospital in year t, R_{it}, is equal to $AC_{i,t-1} (1 + I_g + z \cdot B)$, where $AC_{i,t-1}$ is the ith hospital's average cost in year $t - 1$, I_g is the average rate of cost increase from year $t - 1$ to year t for the hospitals in the group into which the ith hospital falls, z is a number between zero and one, and B is equal to $AC_{it}/AC_{i,t-1} - I_g - 1$ unless this number is negative, in which case B equals zero. In other words, if the ith hospital's rate of cost increase exceeds the group average, the hospital is reimbursed at less than average cost; if its rate of increase is less than the group average, it is reimbursed at more than average cost.[60]

Under this plan the hospital's rate of reimbursement R_{it}/AC_{it}, depends on its rate of average-cost inflation and the mean rate for the group into which it falls. This plan may provide an incentive to cut costs, but it does not distinguish between cost savings achieved by more efficient operation and cost savings achieved by altering product mix.[61] The plan thus might result in unexpected and perhaps undesirable changes in product mix.

Some adjustment for product-mix change might thus be a desirable addition to the plan either to avoid discouraging certain types of product-mix change or to encourage specific types of product-mix change.[62] But does adjustment for product-mix change make any difference? Table 1–15 indicates that it does.

According to the first row of table 1–15, the correlation between the observed rate of inflation and the adjusted rate of inflation never exceeds 0.768 regardless of the adjustment method chosen. The high correlations between inflation rates obtained by various adjustment methods imply that methodological decisions regarding the specification of the cost function and the method of estimation are unimportant in this regard.

In terms of the Waldman plan the first row of table 1–15 implies that

Table 1-15
Correlations between Adjusted Inflation Rates

| | Adjustment Method | | | | | | | | | | | | | |
Adjustment Method	II	III	IV	V	VI	VII	VIII	IX	X	XI	XII	XIII	XIV	XV
I	.716	.694	.733	.712	.757	.727	.743	.692	.747	.745	.684	.675	.768	.744
II		.959	.995	.956	.969	.922	.995	.923	.993	.988	.978	.956	.986	.945
III			.952	.996	.942	.973	.958	.987	.956	.977	.931	.977	.946	.987
IV				.958	.962	.913	.994	.919	.993	.987	.991	.967	.990	.947
V					.937	.966	.959	.986	.958	.978	.946	.990	.952	.991
VI						.963	.959	.906	.955	.954	.928	.918	.943	.917
VII							.916	.959	.912	.935	.877	.931	.898	.950
VIII								.932	.9997	.996	.980	.961	.996	.959
IX									.933	.960	.901	.966	.924	.988
X										.996	.979	.960	.997	.960
XI											.971	.974	.992	.980
XII												.972	.979	.932
XIII													.957	.978
XIV														.959

the relationship between the rate of inflation for an individual hospital and the group mean inflation rate will be altered by the process of adjusting for product-mix change. While this indicates that this process does make a difference in terms of calculating reimbursement rates, table 1–16 indicates that this results primarily from the influence of changing inpatient case-mix. Adjustment for other aspects of product-mix change makes little difference in terms of the relationship between individual hospital and group mean rates of cost inflation.

My findings also have an important implication for the notion of grouping hospitals, namely, that groupings based on costliness of product mix may be unstable. In other words, the relationship between average cost in a particular hospital and group mean average cost is sensitive to changes over time in the hospital's product mix. These conclusions should be appraised in the light of three reservations regarding their validity.

First, I have treated the whole sample as if it were a single group while a detailed reimbursement plan would presumably divide the sample hospitals into a number of groups.[63] It would be interesting to break the sample into more homogeneous groups and recompute the correlations between unadjusted inflation rates and inflation rates adjusted for product-mix change by various methods.

Second, the use of a reimbursement method based on group mean average cost or mean inflation rate would probably reduce the importance of product-mix change by inducing hospitals to conform to the norms of the groups in which they are placed. During the 1961–1964 period the hospitals in the sample were not reimbursed strictly on the basis of group averages, but group averages were used to establish minimum and

Table 1–16
Correlations between Unadjusted and Partially Adjusted
Inflation Rates

Adjustment Method	Correlation Coefficient
XVI	0.979
XVII	0.967
XVIII	0.999
XIX	0.784
XX	0.962
XXI	0.982
XXII	0.968
XXIII	0.999
XXIV	0.830
XXV	0.963

maximum levels of reimbursement.[64] Thus the behavior of the same hospitals over this period should reflect the influence of this grouping. This influence might, of course, have been stronger if the provisions of the reimbursement formula had been different.

Third, changes in inpatient case mix were primarily responsible for the results reported. But since the case-mix data were obtained from a one-day census, part of these changes may be due to differences in sampling errors between the 1961 and 1964 censuses.

Conclusion, Summary, and Implications
for Further Research

Two major conclusions emerge. One is that the impact of product-mix change on observed rates of average-cost inflation over the 1961–1964 period for the sample hospitals was small. This conclusion is somewhat surprising in the light of previous findings and hypotheses concerning recent hospital cost inflation. On the other hand, the extent of product-mix change over this period was not substantial. If product-mix change has been more pronounced since 1964, a similar study of later data might reverse this conclusion. Second, the relationship between the rate of inflation for individual hospitals and the mean rate for the whole sample was found to be sensitive to the process of adjusting for product-mix change. This conclusion is interesting in light of recent developments and proposals in the area of hospital reimbursement.

It was also found that the marginal cost of medical education is substantially in excess of any direct costs associated with medical education programs (see appendix 1A). The primary impact of medical education on costs arose from its impact on average length of patient stay.

The issues raised in this chapter suggest several avenues for further research.

1. Since the impact of product-mix change on inflation was small, it would be interesting to apply the same methodology to data from the post-1964 period. A similar finding for this period would suggest a revision of some current views regarding the nature of hospital cost inflation.

2. The methodology used in this study provides a way to adjust for the impact of product-mix change on cost. Since this methodology could be employed in a reimbursement program that employed adjustments for product-mix differences or changes, it would be interesting to explore the possible details of such programs. In particular, we might consider the possibilities for using such programs to provide incentives to product-mix changes of various kinds, thereby affecting the allocation of resources within the hospital industry.

3. The impact of medical education programs on hospitals merits further study. For example, it would be interesting to obtain samples of cases from teaching hospitals and nonteaching hospitals (or from hospitals with large teaching programs and hospitals with small teaching programs) that are closely matched according to clinical and socioeconomic characteristics and to analyze these case records in detail. Such an analysis could point up the relevant effects of teaching programs on patient care and would either support or refute my findings regarding the costs of medical education. Given the national commitment to expansion of medical education programs, this research seems especially important for informed national policy in this area.

4. The future role of hospitals is a current concern. Should they provide more or less ambulatory care? Should they provide nursing education, or should it be provided by educational institutions? Answers to these questions obviously depend in part on the costs of providing various services by different methods. The cost functions used in the third section make it possible to obtain estimates of the marginal costs of providing services unrelated to inpatient services through the hospital system. To obtain reliable answers to these questions, more research along these lines is necessary.

Notes

1. U.S. Department of Health, Education, and Welfare, *Report of the National Conference on Medical Costs* (Washington, D.C.: U.S. Government Printing Office, 1967); Herbert E. Klarman, "The Increased Cost of Hospital Care," in *The Economics of Health and Medical Care*, Proceedings of the Conference on the Economics of Health and Medical Care, Ann Arbor, May 10–12, 1962 (Ann Arbor, Mich.: University of Michigan, 1964); Herman M. Somers and Anne R. Somers, *Medicare and the Hospitals: Issues and Prospects* (Washington, D.C.: Brookings Institution, 1967), chap. 10; Odin W. Anderson and Duncan Neuhauser, "Rising Costs Are Inherent in Modern Health Care Systems," *Hospitals* 43 (February 1969): 50–52.

2. See Klarman, "Increased Cost of Hospital Care;" Somers and Somers, *Medicare and the Hospitals,* chap. 10; State of Maryland, *Report of the State of Maryland Commission to Study Hospital Costs* (Baltimore, 1964); and State of Minnesota, Legislative Research Committee, Staff Report: *Study on Hospital Rates and Charges* (Minneapolis, 1962).

3. Notice that $\overline{AC}_{i64}$ depends on u_{i64}. If instead u_{i64} were set equal to

zero, we would obtain the odd result that $\overline{AC}_{i64}$ differs from AC_{i64} even if no product-mix change has occurred ($p_{ji64} = p_{ij61}$ for $j = 1, \ldots, n$).

4. If either set of weights yields the same reults, it must be true that $(\overline{AC}_{i64}/AC_{i61}) = (AC_{i64}/\overline{AC}_{i61})$. Since this implies that $(\overline{AC}_{i64}/AC_{i64}) = (AC_{i61}/\overline{AC}_{i61})$, if it were also true that $U_{i61} = U_{i64}$ and $S_{i61} = S_{i64}$, this equality of results would imply a "neutral" shift in the cost function, that is, $F_{61} = K \cdot F_{64}$ where K is a positive constant. The same conclusion would follow if F_{61} and F_{64} were homogeneous of degree zero in U and S and if U and S changed proportionately from 1961 to 1964. Neither of these assumptions about U and S (constancy or proportionate changes) applies to any of the sample hospitals.

5. If more than one capacity utilization measure were used, we would face the difficult problem of defining capacity measures for other products in addition to inpatient care, such as ambulatory patient care or medical education.

6. Since we are treating the hospital as the producer of a composite product, the level of output (the number of units of the composite product actually produced) is measured by the number of units of inpatient care produced. Thus an increase in the units of, say, outpatient care produced represents, in our terminology, a change in the hospital's product mix (in the composite product that it produces) but no change in the level of output.

7. Shorter stays may however be a socially inefficient way to reduce the use of hospital resources since they may impose additional costs on patients and their families. For more discussions of this point and of the relative merits of the case and the patient-day as output measures see Martin S. Feldstein, *Economic Analysis for Health Service Efficiency* (Chicago: Markham Publishing Co., 1968), pp. 24–25. An interesting general discussion of output measurement in hospitals is given in Robert Evans, " 'Behavioural' Cost Functions for Hospitals" (Department of Economics, University of British Columbia, 1970).

8. See, for example, Ralph E. Berry, Jr., "Returns to Scale in the Production of Hospital Services," *Health Services Research* (Summer 1967); and Kong Kyun Ro, "A Statistical Study of Factors Affecting the Unit Cost of Short-Term Hospital Care" (Ph.D. dissertation, Department of Economics, Yale University, 1966).

9. Feldstein's finding that case mix explained 27.5 percent of the variation in cost per case for 177 British hospitals while it explained only 2.1 percent of the variation in cost per patient-week is consistent with this supposition. See Feldstein, *Health Service Efficiency*, p. 23.

For a detailed treatment of the bias due to omission of case-mix variables, see ibid., pp. 64–65.

10. A fourth type of product, medical research, is not relevant to this study since major teaching-research hospitals were excluded from the study sample. Research expenditures by the sample hospitals were minimal. For example, in 1964 only three hospitals reported any research expense at all, and for these three hospitals the mean ratio of research expense to total expense was approximately 0.007.

11. Cross-classifications, such as the age distribution of patients within a particular diagnostic category, were not available to me.

12. For more information on these censuses see "Hospital Service in Southern New York: The Characteristics of the Hospital Population as Shown in Two Censuses of Patients in Short-Term General Care Hospitals on October 20, 1964 and May 10, 1961" (Associated Hospital Service of New York, no date).

13. The case-mix data are subject to two limitations. First, since the censuses were conducted over only one day, the data tend to overstate the percentage of case types that have, on the average, longer lengths of stay. Of course, this difficulty could have been avoided by using the patient-day as the basic unit of output. Second, the lack of cross-classification of patients may be a problem if the cost characteristics of particular case types arise in large part from interactions between age and sex characteristics and diagnostic categories. I shall represent the cost characteristics of a particular case type as the additive effects of sex, age, and diagnosis. If the interaction effects among these three characteristics are small, this representation will be adequate.

14. For an excellent discussion of principal components techniques, see Donald F. Morrison, *Multivariate Statistical Methods* (New York: McGraw-Hill, 1967).

15. More specifically, the first principal component is the linear combination that explains the largest amount of variance in the original variables. The second principal component is the linear combination that explains the largest amount of the variance in the original variables and is uncorrelated with the first principal component, and so on.

16. Notice that table 1–2 lists only twenty-six case-mix variables. One age category, one sex category, and one case type were eliminated from the principal components analysis to avoid singularity of the cross-product matrix of case-mix variables.

17. When the original variables are expressed in dissimilar units, such as, say, dollars and square miles, it is common to extract the principal components from the correlation matrix of the original variables.

18. Analyses in which the identification of components or of factors derived from components is attempted may be found in Mary Lee Ingbar and Lester D. Taylor, *Hospital Costs in Massachusetts* (Cambridge, Mass.: Harvard University Press, 1968), pp. 32–41; Evans, " 'Be-

havioural' Cost Functions''; Ralph E. Berry, Jr., "Product Heterogeneity and Hospital Cost Analysis," *Inquiry* 7 (March 1970): 67–75; and Richard L. Morrill and Robert Earickson, "Hospital Variation and Patient Travel Distance," *Inquiry* 5 (December 1968): 26–34. Other applications of principal components techniques may be found in Feldstein, *Health Service Efficiency*, pp. 19–21, and Ingbar and Taylor, *Hospital Costs in Massachusetts*, pp. 44–45.

19. And even if component identifications were obvious, they still might not represent a stable set of underlying influences. See Irving Lorge and Nathan Morrison, "The Reliability of Principal Components," *Science* 87 (May 27, 1938).

20. We may hypothesize that a disproportionate number of the patients classified under accidents, poisonings, and violence are children.

21. My colleague, J.P. Acton, has suggested a few other patterns roughly consistent with the components; for example, the fourth component may be a positive indicator of older patients with degenerative diseases and a negative indicator of acute (say, heart-attack) patients, and that the third component may distinguish thoracic from subthoracic problems.

22. While factor analysis techniques may be used to obtain orthogonal transformations of the principal components which are more easily identified, there was no reason for employing these techniques here where identification per se is of no particular interest.

23. I had originally planned to include some measure of home care as part of the measurement of ambulatory patient care output, but sufficient data were not available and so I dropped this type of activity from consideration. This omission is probably not very serious; in 1964, for example, only five of the sample hospitals reported any home care expenditures, and for these five hospitals the mean ratio of home care expense to total expense was about 0.003.

24. This distinction is made, for example, in a factor analysis described in Ralph E. Berry, Jr., "An Analysis of Costs in Short-Term General Hospitals: Final Report" (Harvard University, October 1968).

25. For example, a study of the use of emergency room services revealed that only 6 percent of the sample patients had "emergent" problems and only an additional 36 percent had "urgent" problems; see E. Richard Weinerman et al., "Yale Studies in Ambulatory Medical Care, V: Determinants of Use of Hospital Emergency Services," U.S. Public Health Service, *Medical Care in Transition*, vol. 3 (Washington, D.C.: U.S. Government Printing Office, 1967).

26. This figure is given in the consolidated listing of hospitals in the *Directory of Approved Internships and Residencies* (Chicago: American Medical Association, annual). Since this figure is given for the academic

year, the figure for the relevant calendar year was obtained by averaging the figures for the two academic years that overlapped this calendar year.

27. See, for example, Berry, "Returns to Scale," "Product Heterogeneity," "Analysis of Costs," and Karen Davis, "A Theory of Economic Behavior in Non-Profit, Private Hospitals" (Ph.D. dissertation, Rice University, 1969), chap. 4.

28. These data consist of zero-one dummy variables indicating the presence or absence of certain facilities as reported in *Hospitals: Guide Issue* (Chicago: American Hospital Association, annual).

29. ALC and the labor cost component of ATC were computed by adjusting each hospital's wage level to the New York City level. Appendix 1B describes the way in which hospital wage levels were calculated.

30. The case-mix variables correspond to the first twenty-six variables listed in table 1–1. The last three variables in that table were excluded to avoid singularity of the cross-product matrix.

Since the case-mix proportions are based on samples and not on the actual case-mix of the hospital for the year, there is some question about the applicability of OLS in this situation. That is, it might be desirable to estimate the equations in table 1–5 by instrumental variables to allow for errors in the case-mix variables.

31. Recall that a three-way classification of patients was used so that three characteristics are needed to completely describe any single case.

This calculation of the marginal cost is based on the assumption that u takes on its expected value zero.

32. Since identical functional forms were used for the ALC and ANLC equations, addition of the two equations yields an ATC function such as equation 1.9 or 1.10.

33. Thus the coefficients of the estimated ALC equations assume a wage level equal to that of the New York City hospitals in 1964.

34. In other words, the dependent variable in the ALC regressions was $ALC_{i64} \cdot (w_{NYC}/w_i)$ where w_i is the ith hospital's wage index and w_{NYC} is the New York City wage index. Denoting average labor cost adjusted to the 1961 product mix and obtained from the ALC regressions by $\overline{ALC}_{i64}$, and the analogous adjusted average nonlabor cost by $\overline{ANLC}_{i64}$, $\overline{AC}_{i64}$ is obtained from $\overline{AC}_{i64} = \overline{ANLC}_{i64} + \overline{ALC}_{i64} \cdot (w_i/w_{NYC})$.

35. These numbers are slightly sensitive to the fact that each hospital's wage index has been adjusted upward to the New York City level. For example, equation 1.15 implies that as the wage index is adjusted downward, the maximum-cost value of BEDS approaches a value just over 303 while further upward adjustment of the wage index, according to equation 1.13, pushes the maximum-cost size downward toward a value just below 292.

36. The pattern described here has also been found by Ingbar and Taylor, *Hospital Costs in Massachusetts*, pp. 56–59; Berry, "Analysis of Costs," p. 43; and Evans, " 'Behavioural' Cost Functions."

Continuously negative effects were found by Feldstein, *Health Service Efficiency*, p. 75; and Davis, "Theory of Economic Behavior," chap. 4, sec. 2. Feldstein's production function estimates (chap. 4) support the result of continuously negative scale effects although these effects appear to be very small. Production function estimates presented by Davis (chap. 4, sec. 6) indicate either very slightly increasing or very slightly decreasing returns to scale. In short, the evidence from both studies is quite consistent with the hypothesis of zero scale effects (constant returns to scale).

Negative effects followed by positive effects were reported by Berry, "Analysis of Costs," pp. 28–37; and Feldstein, *Health Service Efficiency*, pp. 74–75.

37. Feldstein, *Health Service Efficiency*, pp. 56–60.

38. Ingbar and Taylor (*Hospital Costs in Massachusetts,* p. 111) explain their findings regarding scale effects in a manner similar to the one just outlined.

39. In the equations in table 1–7, BEDS and $BEDS^2$ were included to measure scale effects, and $BEDS^{-1}$ was included to measure product-mix effects. But the results indicate the same pattern of scale effects as before. In table 1–8 the sign of $BEDS^{-1}$ is always positive. Since this would imply product-mix effects that are negatively related to size, it might be more sensible to interpret $BEDS^{-1}$ as measuring scale effects that are always negative but approach zero as size increases. BEDS and Log(BEDS) might be interpreted as measuring product-mix effects. Their coefficients, which imply increasing cost as size increases until a maximum of about 300 beds and then decreasing costs, are roughly consistent with this interpretation. But the *t*-values for all the relevant coefficients are so small that none of these results can be taken very seriously.

40. Feldstein, *Health Service Efficiency*; Ingbar and Taylor, *Hospital Costs in Massachusetts*.

41. In attempting to distinguish between these two types of effect, several average-cost functions were estimated with average length of inpatient stay included in the list of independent variables. Other studies in which this variable has been used to adjust for product-mix differences are Evans, " 'Behavioural' Cost Functions," and Berry, "Product Heterogeneity." In my analysis, however, including length of stay as an independent variable did not radically alter the coefficients for BEDS and $BEDS^2$.

42. While this might not be true if the change from the 350-bed

hospital to the 450-bed hospital is also a change from a "community" hospital to a major center of medical education and research, the latter type of institution has been excluded from this sample.

43. If BEDS^{-1} is an adequate substitute for BEDS and BEDS^2, we expect that adding BEDS and BEDS^2 to equations 1.25 and 1.27 would not change our results significantly. More formally, we expect that the two-element vector whose elements are the coefficient of BEDS and the coefficient of BEDS^2 would not be significantly different from a vector of zeroes when these variables are added to equations 1.25 and 1.27. This may be tested by computing the relevant F-statistics from equations 1.25 and 1.17 and from equations 1.27 and 1.18. These F-values, 0.81 and 0.13 respectively, are not significantly different from zero at even minimal levels of significance.

44. Since BEDS^{-1} is interpreted as a product-mix variable, pure scale changes will not affect average cost through the impact of this variable. That is, interpreting BEDS^{-1} as a product-mix variable implies that pure scale changes will not affect BEDS^{-1}. A pure scale increase will only reduce FLOW, for a given number of cases, thereby increasing average cost since the coefficient of Log(FLOW) is negative. Thus the cost-minimizing scale is zero.

45. Since equation 1.25 implies an optimal rate of 57.7 while equation 1.27 implies an optimal rate of 66.9, the optimal rate implied by their sum is somewhat sensitive to the choice of a wage index used to adjust labor costs.

46. Feldstein, in his study of British hospitals, obtained a much lower optimal flow rate of 32.3 when he estimated an average-cost function similar to those under consideration, but this optimal rate was also near the upper end of the range of observed flow rates. See Feldstein, *Health Service Efficiency*, pp. 74, 130.

47. We expect the demand for hospital care to be inelastic with respect to price but not completely inelastic. Such a result was reported by Gerald Rosenthal, *The Demand for General Hospital Facilities* (Chicago: American Hospital Association, 1964). A recent study by Karen Davis reports evidence that this demand is in fact price elastic ("Production and Cost Function Estimation for Non-Profit Hospitals, Rice University, n.d.).

48. Since the sample is not very large, the fact that the OLS estimates are not consistent while the instrumental variables estimates are does not argue strongly for use of the latter estimates. If in fact FLOW and FLOW^2 are endogenous variables, neither set of estimates is unbiased.

The instrumental variables estimates may still be inconsistent, since it is not clear that the case-flow group numbers can be regarded as truly exogenous. But the relationship between these numbers and the error term in the cost function is much weaker than that between the error term and the actual values of FLOW and $FLOW^2$. At the very least, then, the coefficient estimates obtained by the instrumental-variables procedure should be much less asymptotically biased than the OLS estimates.

The simpler procedure, used by Feldstein (*Health Service Efficiency,* pp. 80–81), of using the case-flow group numbers as instruments performed very poorly because very high correlations between the fitted values of FLOW and $FLOW^2$ resulted from this choice of instruments.

49. For a description of the test, see Feldstein, *Health Service Efficiency,* appendix 2A. In his estimation of cross-sectional cost functions, Feldstein found evidence of substantial heteroskedasticity.

50. Ibid.

51. Given the low t-values on the coefficients of NEDUC this figure should be taken with a grain of salt. But the findings of other studies suggest that a small negative marginal cost for nursing education is a reasonable result. For example, Ingbar and Whitney found that each dollar spent on nursing education reduced costs in the nursing service department alone by $0.90. See Mary Lee Ingbar and Barbara J. Whitney, "Differences in the Costs of Nursing Service" (Harvard University, 1964). If nursing education also reduces costs in other departments (such as by replacing other types of employees by student nurses), the total impact of nursing education on cost will be negative. Of course, my findings suggest a net negative impact on both labor and nonlabor costs. The negative impact on nonlabor costs implies the substitution of relatively cheap nursing student labor for nonlabor inputs.

52. Another possible result, that the hospital's facilities are used less intensively, would not affect the estimated marginal cost since FLOW and $FLOW^2$ correct for differences in the rate of capacity utilization.

53. The means for MEDUC, ATC, and LOS are calculated from the seventy-three hospitals whose rates of inflation are studied in the fourth section of this chapter rather than from all seventy-six hospitals included in the sample for purposes of estimating cost functions.

54. The number of hospitals remaining in the same size class is obtained by summing the diagonal elements of table 1–13. The number of hospitals that moved up two or more size classes is obtained by summing all elements two columns or more to the right of the diagonal.

55. See note 39.

56. The increase in COMP 1 must reflect, at least in part, the well-known decline in the use of obstetric services.

57. See, for example, *Report of the State of Maryland Commission to Study Hospital Costs* (1964), p. 1.

58. The notion of grouping hospitals has already been put into practice. For example, the Associated Hospital Service of New York groups

hospitals according to size, location, and scope of services for purposes of computing reimbursement rates. See "Member Hospital Reimbursement Formula: Effective January 1, 1970," mimeographed (Associated Hospital Service of New York, 1969).

59. See Saul Waldman, " 'Average Increase in Costs': An Incentive-Reimbursement Formula for Hospitals," *Reimbursement Incentives for Hospitals and Medical Care: Objectives and Alternatives,* Research Report No. 26, Office of Research and Statistics, Social Security Administration (Washington, D.C.: U.S. Government Printing Office, 1968).

60. Ibid., p. 43.

61. The popular notion of the hospital as a public utility that "takes all comers" is incorrect. In the short run hospitals can and do practice selective admissions policies. (This is more prevalent, however, among proprietary hospitals than among voluntary hospitals.) In the long run hospitals can change the range of facilities and services that they offer and change the specialty composition of the members of the medical staff. In other words, hospitals can alter their product mix in both the short run and the long run.

62. The question of what kinds of product-mix change are desirable has been the subject of much recent debate. There is, for example, much disagreement over whether hospitals should in the future continue to expand their role as providers of primary (ambulatory) care.

63. According to the Associated Hospital Service's formula, the sample hospitals fall into six different groups ("Member Hospital Reimbursement Formula").

64. In particular, no hospital was reimbursed at a level greater than the level that would be paid to a hospital whose per diem reimbursable expense exceeded the group average by 15 percent. Provided that a hospital satisfied certain other requirements, it could not be reimbursed at a level less than that given to a hospital whose per diem reimbursable expense was 15 percent less than the group average. See *Member Hospital Reimbursement Formula: Review Committee Decisions and Administrative Interpretations through December 31, 1965* (Associated Hospital Service of New York, no date), pp. 41–46.

Appendix 1A
Further Results on the
Costs of Medical
Education

The purpose of this appendix is to analyze in further detail the impact of medical education on costs. After adjusting for the effects of capacity-utilization differences (by including FLOW and FLOW^2 in equations 1.35, 1.36, and 1.37), I found that almost all the impact of MEDUC on ATC (= ALC + ANLC) appears to result from its impact on LOS. But if MEDUC influences ATC by affecting the rate at which patients move through the treatment process, as I have hypothesized, it probably also affects capacity utilization (as measured by FLOW). Stated more simply, if MEDUC influences LOS it should also influence FLOW, since

$$FLOW = 366 \times (\text{occupancy rate})/LOS \qquad (1A.1)$$

The constant in the formula for FLOW is 366 rather than 365 because 1964 was a leap year.

To measure the magnitude of the effect of MEDUC on FLOW, the following equation was estimated by OLS; all other equations in this appendix were also estimated by OLS.

$$
\begin{aligned}
FLOW = 39.69 &- 2{,}751 \text{ MEDUC} + 81.16 \text{ NEDUC} - 0.4857 \text{ AMB} \\
(6.31) \quad &(3.23) \qquad\qquad (0.34) \qquad\qquad (1.00) \\[4pt]
&- 315.1 \text{ BEDS}^{-1} - 0.3500 \text{ COMP 1} + 0.3086 \text{ COMP 2} \\
&(2.60) \qquad\quad (5.96) \qquad\qquad\;\; (3.80) \\[4pt]
&- 0.0136 \text{ COMP 1} + 0.0392 \text{ COMP 2} + 0.0192 \text{ COMP 5} \\
&(0.11) \qquad\qquad (0.76) \qquad\qquad\;\; (0.16) \\[4pt]
&- 0.3804 \text{ COMP 6} - 0.3887 \text{ COMP 7} \qquad\qquad (1A.2) \\
&(2.67) \qquad\qquad (1.93)
\end{aligned}
$$

$R^2 = 0.58$

The coefficient of MEDUC is, as expected, negative and significant. Medical education both increases LOS and reduces FLOW. Using mean values of 34.29 and 0.00075 for FLOW and MEDUC respectively, the elasticity of FLOW with respect to MEDUC according to equation 1A.2 is -0.060. These means and others mentioned in the appendix apply to all seventy-six hospitals.

Equation 1.37 displayed a positive effect of MEDUC on LOS when FLOW and FLOW² were held constant. But equation 1A.1 indicates that if FLOW is constant and LOS increases, occupancy rate (OCC) must also increase. To check this result and to estimate the elasticity of LOS with respect to MEDUC when FLOW and FLOW² are not held constant, the equations shown in table 1A–1 were estimated.

As indicated by equations 1A.5 and 1A.6, MEDUC does have a positive effect on OCC; the coefficients of MEDUC in equations 1A.5 and

Table 1A–1
Regressions of LOS, Log(LOS), OCC, Log(OCC) and Log(FLOW) on Product-Mix Variables

		Equation Number			
Dependent Variable	1A.3 LOS	1A.4 Log (LOS)	1A.5 OCC	1A.6 Log (OCC)	1A.7 Log (FLOW)
MEDUC	1153 (5.7)	118.2 (6.32)	22.47 (1.85)	29.07 (1.74)	−89.15 (3.58)
NEDUC	−53.17 (0.95)	−4.178 (0.81)	0.3292 (0.10)	0.4642 (0.10)	4.643 (0.68)
AMB	0.0859 (0.74)	−0.0095 (0.89)	−0.0144 (2.07)	−0.0193 (2.02)	−0.0098 (0.69)
BEDS⁻¹	23.53 (0.82)	1.188 (.45)	−5.964 (3.46)	−9.040 (3.81)	−10.23 (2.89)
COMP 1	0.1078 (7.72)	0.0111 (8.61)	−0.0004 (0.45)	−0.0003 (0.29)	−0.0115 (6.66)
COMP 2	−0.0704 (3.65)	−0.0083 (4.67)	0.0008 (0.67)	0.0006 (0.35)	0.0089 (3.75)
COMP 3	−0.0170 (.58)	−0.0026 (0.97)	−0.0026 (1.49)	−0.0044 (1.80)	−0.0017 (0.48)
COMP 4	−0.0616 (2.12)	−0.0051 (1.89)	−0.0002 (0.12)	0.0002 (0.07)	0.0053 (1.47)
COMP 5	0.0084 (0.29)	−0.0014 (0.50)	−0.0007 (0.41)	−0.0014 (0.56)	0.00005 (0.001)
COMP 6	0.0860 (2.54)	0.0095 (3.03)	−0.0003 (0.15)	−0.0008 (0.30)	−0.0103 (2.47)
COMP 7	0.1055 (2.53)	0.0105 (2.73)	−0.0003 (0.12)	−0.0005 (0.14)	−0.0110 (2.15)
Constant	7.900 (5.28)	2.160 (15.61)	0.9503 (10.58)	0.0155 (0.13)	3.758 (20.39)
R^2	0.67	0.72	0.28	0.31	0.61
Elasticity wrt MEDUC	0.100	0.089	0.022	0.022	−0.067

1A.6 are significant at the 5 percent level. But the elasticity of OCC with respect to MEDUC is substantially less than the corresponding elasticity for LOS.[1] Equation 1A.7 indicates an estimate of the elasticity of FLOW with respect to MEDUC that is similar to that derived from equation 1A.2.[2]

In summary, equations 1A.2 and 1A.7 clearly indicate that medical education has a negative impact on the rate of capacity utilization in the sample hospitals and that this arises primarily from the impact of MEDUC on LOS. And if this impact is allowed for, the estimated marginal cost of an additional year of physician education will be different from the estimate of this marginal cost derived from equations 1.35 and 1.36, since FLOW and $FLOW^2$ were included in these equations. To obtain an estimate of marginal cost that includes the cost effect of the impact of MEDUC on FLOW, the following regression was estimated:

$$ATC = 286.5 + 42{,}775\ MEDUC - 2804.5\ NEDUC + 8.0731\ AMB$$
$$\quad (4.49)\quad (4.96)\qquad\qquad (1.18)\qquad\qquad (1.64)$$

$$\qquad + 2.2121\ COMP\ 1 - 3.307\ COMP\ 2 + 1.8346\ COMP\ 3$$
$$\qquad\quad (3.71)\qquad\qquad (4.02)\qquad\qquad (1.46)$$

$$\qquad - 1.6547\ COMP\ 4 + 0.5625\ COMP\ 5 + 2.6715\ COMP\ 6$$
$$\qquad\quad (1.33)\qquad\qquad (0.45)\qquad\qquad (1.85)$$

$$\qquad + 4.2666\ COMP\ 7 - 741.05\ BEDS^{-1}\qquad\qquad (1.A8)$$
$$\qquad\quad (2.40)\qquad\qquad (0.60)$$

$$R^2 = 0.67$$

The coefficient of MEDUC indicates that the marginal cost of an additional year of physician education is almost \$43,000. This is about \$16,000 greater than the estimate obtained from equations 1.35 and 1.36. Thus when the impact of medical education on the rate of capacity utilization is allowed for, the estimated marginal cost of physician education increases substantially.[3]

The linear relationship between ATC and MEDUC in equation 1A.8 implies the assumption that the marginal cost of physician education is constant. To test this assumption, a number of equations (reported in tables 1A–2 and 1A–3) were estimated. Four additional variables are included in these equations.

D1 = A dummy variable equal to one if MEDUC is positive and equal to zero if MEDUC is equal to zero

D2 = a dummy variable equal to one if $MEDUC > 0.0016$ and equal to zero if $MEDUC \leq 0.0016$

D3 = a variable equal to one divided by the number of cases if MEDUC is positive and equal to zero if MEDUC is equal to zero

D4 = a variable equal to one divided by the number of cases if MEDUC > 0.0016 and equal to zero if MEDUC ≤ 0.0016.[4]

Table 1A–2
Tests on the Form of the Relationship between Average Cost per Case and Medical Education
(t-values in parentheses)

	Equation Number					
Dependent Variable	*1A.9* ATC	*1A.10* ATC	*1A.11* ATC	*1A.12* ATC	*1A.13* ATC	*1A.14* ATC
MEDUC			25,084 (1.08)	45,646 (2.95)	41,325 (4.30)	3,607.2 (0.12)
NEDUC	−1,014.1 (0.38)	−1,716.2 (0.68)	−2,475.3 (1.02)	−2,969.4 (1.22)	−2,901.1 (1.20)	−2,522 (1.04)
AMB	19.303 (3.98)	15.31 (3.20)	9.2732 (1.80)	7.2426 (1.37)	7.72 (1.52)	9.0997 (1.76)
BEDS^{-1}	−165.97 (0.11)	−631.29 (0.44)	−1,057.2 (0.82)	−511.89 (0.38)	−556.57 (0.42)	−681.2 (0.51)
COMP 1	2.2657 (3.30)	2.4262 (3.73)	2.2154 (3.71)	2.2169 (3.58)	2.2482 (3.70)	2.3491 (3.85)
COMP 2	−3.3851 (3.55)	−3.2133 (3.56)	−3.3684 (4.06)	−3.2669 (3.83)	−3.2495 (3.85)	−3.2173 (3.83)
COMP 3	1.9952 (1.39)	1.4883 (1.09)	1.6138 (126)	1.9835 (1.52)	1.9002 (1.49)	1.6484 (1.28)
COMP 4	−1.6772 (1.19)	−1.7483 (1.31)	−1.7768 (1.42)	−1.6217 (1.29)	−1.6388 (1.31)	−1.8314 (1.46)
COMP 5	1.4484 (1.03)	0.8917 (0.67)	0.5645 (0.45)	0.602 (0.48)	0.5895 (0.47)	0.6637 (0.53)
COMP 6	2.3157 (1.41)	2.9744 (1.90)	2.8107 (1.93)	2.5507 (1.72)	2.6380 (1.81)	2.8176 (1.93)
COMP 7	2.3004 (1.15)	3.3299 (1.73)	4.3807 (2.45)	4.1473 (2.26)	4.1438 (2.28)	4.0419 (2.23)
D1	54.847 (2.14)	29.749 (1.16)		8.6895 (0.34)	8.883 (0.35)	32.078 (1.04)
D2		75.704 (2.94)		−13.913 (0.36)		
D2·MEDUC			15,863 (0.82)			30,425 (1.28)
Constant	228.6 (3.04)	272.8 (3.76)	299.4 (4.55)	276.2 (4.03)	279.1 (4.13)	284.3 (4.22)
R^2	0.58	0.63	0.68	0.67	0.67	0.68

Table 1A–3
Further Tests on the Form of the Relationship between Average Cost per Case and Medical Education
(t-values in parentheses)

Dependent Variable	Equation Number			
	1A.15 ATC	1A.16 ATC	1A.17 ATC	1A.18 ATC
MEDUC			16,790 (0.97)	37,558 (3.81)
NEDUC	−206.03 (0.08)	−205.79 (0.09)	−1272.8 (0.50)	−2592.5 (1.09)
AMB	14.274 (2.71)	7.3593 (1.46)	6.1841 (1.19)	6.1455 (1.17)
BEDS^{-1}	−25.535 (0.02)	−770.26 (0.60)	−627.0 (0.48)	−297.40 (0.23)
COMP 1	2.1318 (3.26)	2.1685 (3.68)	2.2019 (3.73)	2.2358 (3.76)
COMP 2	−3.3054 (3.62)	−3.1850 (3.87)	−3.1672 (3.84)	−3.1698 (3.81)
COMP 3	1.9739 (1.43)	1.1993 (0.95)	1.4701 (1.14)	1.9635 (1.56)
COMP 4	−1.722 (1.26)	−1.9491 (1.58)	−1.8324 (1.48)	−1.6416 (1.32)
COMP 5	1.0846 (0.80)	0.30135 (0.24)	0.3317 (0.27)	0.5295 (0.43)
COMP 6	2.2478 (1.42)	2.8879 (2.01)	2.8004 (1.94)	2.5612 (1.77)
COMP 7	2.2022 (1.14)	3.5574 (2.01)	3.8260 (2.13)	3.8809 (2.15)
D3	585,890 (3.05)	311,260 (1.68)	244,260 (1.23)	217,590 (1.09)
D4		749,710 (4.00)	483,140 (1.45)	
Constant	243.2 (3.44)	313.6 (4.75)	302.4 (4.51)	274.2 (4.24)
R^2	0.60	0.68	0.69	0.68

The specification of equation 1A.9 implies that there is a constant difference in ATC between hospitals with no medical education and hospitals with some medical education. This difference is measured by the coefficient of D1. The notion being tested here is that when a hospital establishes residency or internship programs it somehow "does things differently" (and that this difference results in a higher cost per case). If this notion is correct, the omission of D1 from equation 1A.8 biases the estimate of the marginal cost of physician education upward. Equation

1A.10 includes the assumption that hospitals with relatively more medical education do things differently from hospitals with relatively little medical education. Thus hospitals are divided into three groups: (1) those with no medical education, (2) those with relatively little medical education, and (3) those with relatively more medical education. The constant difference in ATC between groups 1 and 2 is measured by the coefficient of D1 while the corresponding difference between groups 2 and 3 is measured by the coefficient of D2.[5] Both equations imply that the marginal cost of medical education is zero. We ignore the possibility, in equation 1A.10, of a hospital's moving between groups. Equations 1A.12 and 1A.13 imply that while these constant intergroup differences in ATC exist (and are measured by the coefficients of D1 and D2), there is also a constant marginal cost of additional medical education (measured by the coefficient of MEDUC). Equation 1A.14 implies a constant difference in ATC between hospitals with no medical education and hospitals with some medical education and a difference in the hospital cost of additional medical education between the hospitals in group 2 and those in group 3 (as measured by the coefficient of D2 · MEDUC). Equation 1A.11 eliminates the constant difference in ATC and only assumes the difference in marginal cost.

Comparing equations 1A.9 and 1A.10 with 1A.12 and 1A.13, we find that the coefficients of D1 and D2 become extremely insignificant in the latter two equations. That is, the assumption of constant intergroup differences in ATC is not supported by the data when we permit the marginal cost of medical education to be nonzero. The relatively low t-value (1.04) of the coefficient of D1 in equation 1A.14 also indicates that the constant-difference assumption works poorly when intergroup differences in marginal cost are allowed for. Also the estimated marginal cost of medical education in equations 1A.12 and 1A.13 is almost identical to the estimate from equation 1A.9. Finally, the assumption of differences of marginal cost does not perform very well. The modest t-values for the coefficients of MEDUC and D2· MEDUC in 1A.11 and 1A.14 are obviously the result of strong collinearity between these variables.

In the next set of regressions we examine the possibility that the estimate of the marginal cost of medical education is biased upward because equation 1A.8 implies that the fixed cost of medical education is zero. The coefficient of D3 in 1A.15 is the estimate of the fixed cost of medical education on the assumption that the marginal cost is zero.[6] In equation 1A.16 the coefficients of D3 measure the fixed difference in total cost between group 1 and group 2 hospitals while the coefficient of D4 measures the fixed difference in total costs between group 2 and group 3 hospitals. Equations 1A.17 and 1A.18 maintain these assumptions about fixed differences in total cost while dropping the assumption that the

Table 1A–4
***F*-Tests on Coefficients of D1, D2, D3, D4, D2·MEDUC**

Equations Compared	Variables	Value of F(2,62)
1A.8, 1A.12	D1, D2	0.12
1A.8, 1A.14	D1, D2·MEDUC	0.88
1A.8, 1A.17	D3, D4	1.66

marginal cost is zero. Equation 1A.18 indicates that the assumption of fixed differences in total costs between hospitals in group 1 and hospitals in groups 2 and 3 works moderately well at best. Also it only lowers the estimate of the marginal cost by about $5,000. Slightly better results are obtained in equation 1A.17, where fixed total-cost differences are assumed between groups 2 and 3 as well. Here the estimated marginal cost is reduced substantially, but collinearity between D3, D4, and MEDUC results in relatively low *t*-values for their coefficients.

Finally, by comparing equation 1A.8 with equations in 1A–2 and 1A–3 we may test the hypothesis that the coefficients of the additional variables included in these equations, when taken together, are different from zero. The results of these tests are reported in table 1A–4.[7] Since an *F*-value with two and sixty degrees of freedom must exceed 2.39 to be significantly different from zero at the 90 percent level, the values reported in table 1A–4 do not indicate that the coefficients in question are different from zero at conventional levels of significance.

In summary, the form of the relationship between ATC and MEDUC in equation 1A.8 seems to fit the data about as well as the more complicated forms implied by the equations in tables 1A–2 and 1A–3. Thus these equations do not provide strong evidence that the estimated marginal cost in equation 1A.8 is seriously in error.

Notes

1. In equations 1A.3 and 1A.5, these elasticities are calculated at means, for LOS and OCC, of 8.635 and 0.769 respectively. Equation 1A.4 is derived from the equation LOS = exp $(a_0 + a_1 \text{ MEDUC} + \ldots + u)$, where u is an error term. The elasticity of LOS with respect to MEDUC, derived from this equation is equal to a_1 MEDUC and was evaluated, in 1A–1, at the mean (0.00075) of MEDUC. Similar comments apply for equations 1A.6 and 1A.7.

2. Equations 1A.3 and 1A.5 or 1A.4 and 1A.6 may also be used to derive estimates of this elasticity by using equation 1A.1.

3. Several other interesting features of equation 1A.8 should also be noted. While the estimated marginal cost of an ambulatory patient visit (the coefficient of AMB) is fairly close to the estimate derived from equations 1.35 and 1.36, the estimated negative marginal cost of a year of nursing education (the coefficient of NEDUC) has increased substantially in absolute value. (This coefficient, however, is only slightly larger than its standard error.) This change arises from the positive (but insignificant) effect of NEDUC on FLOW. Also, the coefficient of $BEDS^{-1}$ is much smaller (in absolute value) and less significant in 1A.8 than in 1.35 and 1.36. This is due to the negative impact of $BEDS^{-1}$ on FLOW as shown in equations 1A.2 and 1A.7.

4. Of the seventy-six hospitals studied, twenty-nine had positive values for MEDUC. Of these twenty-nine, fifteen had values for MEDUC that exceeded 0.0016.

5. The groups referred to here are not the same as the groups mentioned in Appendix B of this Chapter.

6. Since D3 is equal to one over the number of cases, multiplying equation 1A.15 by the number of cases yields a total-cost equation and D3 becomes a one-zero dummy variable indicating the presence of medical education.

7. The reported t-values may be used to test the significance of these coefficients taken individually.

Appendix 1B
Description of Data

Almost all the data used in this study were provided by the associated Hospital Service of New York, which is the Blue Cross organization serving the counties in New York State in which the sample hospitals are located.[1] Data on inpatient case mix were collected in two one-day censuses. Data on costs, nursing education, ambulatory care, bed complement, and inpatient discharges were taken from the Financial and Statistical Reports for the years 1961 and 1964 which each hospital was required to submit to the Associated Hospital Service. The parts of these reports from which data were drawn appear in tables 1B–1 to 1B–6.[2]

The reports submitted by member hospitals are subjected to a two-part auditing procedure. First, a cursory audit is performed by the Associated Hospital Service; then the report is audited more thoroughly by one of several accounting firms regularly employed by the Associated Hospital Service for this purpose. This auditing process thus results in a highly reliable body of information.

The sample hospitals are located in the following counties: Nassau, Suffolk, Bronx, New York, Kings, Richmond, Queens, Westchester, Putnam, Rockland, Delaware, Ulster, Dutchess, Columbia, Orange, Greene, and Sullivan. Twenty-nine of the seventy-three hospitals are located in New York City. Table 1B–7 presents further information on the characteristics of these hospitals.

To exclude major teaching and research centers, all hospitals classified in 1967 as in group 1 or group 2 by the Associated Hospital Service were excluded. The definition of group 1 hospitals is

Accredited voluntary general hospitals rendering at least 200,000 patient days annually (exclusive of newborn days) that meet the following requirements:
1. Full-time physicians serving as residents under an American Medical Association approved residency training program covering at least thirteen different specialties of which ten must be clinical specialties including internal medicine and surgery.
2. A professional nursing school or an affiliation which requires the regular training of professional nursing students on at least two clinical services under an agreement with a college or university offering a degree course in nursing.
3. Full-time physicians serving as interns under an AMA approved internship program.
4. A licensed outpatient department and an emergency service.[3]

Table 1B–1

Report for Year Ended December 31, 1961: Statement of Expenses for Voluntary Hospitals

Expenses	Salaries	Other than Salaries	Total
Expenses for computation			
1. Administration and general	$ _____	$ _____	$ _____
2. Interest expense	$ _____	$ _____	$ _____
3. Operation of plant	$ _____	$ _____	$ _____
4. Maintenance of plant	$ _____	$ _____	$ _____
5. Maintenance of personnel	$ _____	$ _____	$ _____
6. Housekeeping	$ _____	$ _____	$ _____
7. Laundry	$ _____	$ _____	$ _____
8. Linen	$ _____	$ _____	$ _____
9. Raw food	$ _____	$ _____	$ _____
10. Other dietary expenses	$ _____	$ _____	$ _____
11. Medical records	$ _____	$ _____	$ _____
12. Social service	$ _____	$ _____	$ _____
13. Interns and residents	$ _____	$ _____	$ _____
14. Central supply	$ _____	$ _____	$ _____
15. Medical and surgical expense	$ _____	$ _____	$ _____
16. Nursing service	$ _____	$ _____	$ _____
17. School of nursing	$ _____	$ _____	$ _____
18. Pharmacy	$ _____	$ _____	$ _____
19. Operation and recovery rooms	$ _____	$ _____	$ _____
20. Anesthesia	$ _____	$ _____	$ _____
21. Delivery rooms	$ _____	$ _____	$ _____
22. Radiology, diagnostic	$ _____	$ _____	$ _____
23. Radiology, therapeutic	$ _____	$ _____	$ _____
24. Laboratory	$ _____	$ _____	$ _____
25. Electrocardiograph	$ _____	$ _____	$ _____
26. Physical therapy	$ _____	$ _____	$ _____
27. Oxygen therapy	$ _____	$ _____	$ _____
28. Occupational therapy	$ _____	$ _____	$ _____
29. Blood and blood plasma	$ _____	$ _____	$ _____
30. Ambulance	$ _____	$ _____	$ _____
31. Outpatient clinics	$ _____	$ _____	$ _____
32. Emergency service	$ _____	$ _____	$ _____
33. Other patient care services (specify)	$ _____	$ _____	$ _____
34.	$ _____	$ _____	$ _____
35.	$ _____	$ _____	$ _____
36.	$ _____	$ _____	$ _____
37.	$ _____	$ _____	$ _____
38.	$ _____	$ _____	$ _____
39. Public restaurants	$ _____	$ _____	$ _____
40. Gift shop	$ _____	$ _____	$ _____
41. Total: Post to schedule A, line 7	$ _____	$ _____	$ _____
42. Research	$ _____	$ _____	$ _____
43. NYC custodian	$ _____	$ _____	$ _____
44. Collection fees	$ _____	$ _____	$ _____
45. Appeal for funds	$ _____	$ _____	$ _____
46. Extraordinary repairs and maintenance	$ _____	$ _____	$ _____
47. Supervision of interns and residents	$ _____	$ _____	$ _____
48. Other (specify)	$ _____	$ _____	$ _____
49.	$ _____	$ _____	$ _____
50. Replacement of equipment	$ _____		
51. Depreciation of buildings	$ _____	$ _____	$ _____
52. Depreciation of equipment	$ _____	$ _____	$ _____

Table 1B–2
Report for Year Ended December 31, 1961: Inpatient Statistical Data

Data	Adults and Children (Col. 1)	Premature Infants (Col. 2)	Newborn Infants (Col. 3)
Accommodation data			
Discharges			
1. Private	___	___	___
2. Semi-private	___	___	___
3. Ward	___	___	___
4. Total	___	___	___
Patient days			
5. Private	___	___	___
6. Semiprivate	___	___	___
7. Ward	___	___	___
8. Total	___	___	___
Financial status data			
Discharges			
9. Pay or part pay	___	___	___
10. Public charges	___	___	___
11. Free patients	___	___	___
12. Total	___	___	___
Patient days			
13. Pay or part pay	___	___	___
14. Public charges	___	___	___
15. Free patients	___	___	___
16. Total	___	___	___
Miscellaneous			
17. Number of deaths included in discharges	___	___	___
18. Census on last day of year	___	___	___

Class of service data	Admissions	Patient Days
19. Medical-surgical	___	___
20. Pediatrics	___	___
21. Obstetrics	___	___
22. Psychiatric	___	___
23. Other (specify)	___	___
24. Total	___	___

Bed complement	Private	Semiprivate	Ward (Four Beds or Less)	Ward (More Than Four Beds)	All
Adults and children					
25. Medical-surgical	___	___	___	___	___
26. Pediatrics	___	___	___	___	___
27. Obstetrics	___	___	___	___	___
28. Psychiatric	___	___	___	___	___
29.	___	___	___	___	___
30. Total	___	___	___	___	___
31. Occupancy, %	___	___	___	___	___
Newborn bassinets					
32. Premature infants	___	___	___	___	___
33. Newborn infants	___	___	___	___	___
34. Total	___	___	___	___	___

Table 1B–3
Report for Year Ended December 31, 1961: Miscellaneous Statistical Data

Hospital Personnel	Full-Time	Part-Time Number of Employees	Part-Time Weekly Hours Worked
1. Administrative and general			
2. Operation and maintenance of plant			
3. Housekeeping			
4. Laundry and sewing room			
5. Dietary			
6. Clinicians and medical chiefs			
7. Interns and residents			
8. Registered nurses			
9. Licensed practical nurses			
10. Orderlies, aides, and attendants			
11. Student nurses			
12. Social service			
13. Medical records			
14. Pharmacy			
15. Central supply			
16. Operating and recovery rooms			
17. Delivery rooms			
18. Radiology, diagnostic			
19. Radiology, therapeutic			
20. Laboratory			
21. Electrocardiograph			
22. Physical therapy			
23. Oxygen therapy			
24. Occupational therapy			
25. Blood bank			
26. Ambulance			
27. Outpatient clinics			
28. Emergency service			
29. All other employees			
30. Total employees			

Outpatient statistics	Number of Visits	Number of Different Individuals
36. Clinic		
37. Emergency department		
38. Private ambulatory patients		

Table 1B–4

Report for Year Ended December 31, 1964: Statement of Expenses for Voluntary Hospitals

Expenses	Salaries	Other Than Salaries	Total
Expenses for Computation			
1. Administration and general	$ _____	$ _____	$ _____
2. Employee health and welfare	$ _____	$ _____	$ _____
3. Interest expense	$ _____	$ _____	$ _____
4. Operation and maintenance of plant	$ _____	$ _____	$ _____
5. Laundry and linen	$ _____	$ _____	$ _____
6. Housekeeping	$ _____	$ _____	$ _____
7. Dietary, raw food	$ _____	$ _____	$ _____
8. Dietary, other	$ _____	$ _____	$ _____
9. Employee's cafeteria	$ _____	$ _____	$ _____
10. Maintance of personnel	$ _____	$ _____	$ _____
11. Medical records	$ _____	$ _____	$ _____
12. Social service	$ _____	$ _____	$ _____
13. Interns and residents	$ _____	$ _____	$ _____
14. Medical supplies and expense	$ _____	$ _____	$ _____
15. Nursing service	$ _____	$ _____	$ _____
16. School of nursing	$ _____	$ _____	$ _____
17. Pharmacy	$ _____	$ _____	$ _____
18. Other (specify)	$ _____	$ _____	$ _____
19. Intensive nursing care	$ _____	$ _____	$ _____
20. Operating and recovery rooms	$ _____	$ _____	$ _____
22. Anesthesia	$ _____	$ _____	$ _____
22. Delivery rooms	$ _____	$ _____	$ _____
23. Radiology, diagnostic	$ _____	$ _____	$ _____
24. Radiology, therapeutic	$ _____	$ _____	$ _____
25. Laboratory	$ _____	$ _____	$ _____
26. Electrocardiograph	$ _____	$ _____	$ _____
27. Physical therapy	$ _____	$ _____	$ _____
28. Oxygen therapy	$ _____	$ _____	$ _____
29. Blood and blood plasma	$ _____	$ _____	$ _____
30. Other (specify)	$ _____	$ _____	$ _____
31.	$ _____	$ _____	$ _____
32.	$ _____	$ _____	$ _____
33. Ambulance	$ _____	$ _____	$ _____
34. Outpatient clinics	$ _____	$ _____	$ _____
35. Emergency service	$ _____	$ _____	$ _____
36. Home care department	$ _____	$ _____	$ _____
37. Other (specify)	$ _____	$ _____	$ _____
38.	$ _____	$ _____	$ _____
39. Total: Post to schedule A, line 7	$ _____	$ _____	$ _____
40. Public restaurants	$ _____	$ _____	$ _____
41. Gift shop	$ _____	$ _____	$ _____
42. Research	$ _____	$ _____	$ _____
43. Collection fees	$ _____	$ _____	$ _____
44. Appeal for funds	$ _____	$ _____	$ _____
45. Extraordinary repairs and maintenance	$ _____	$ _____	$ _____
46. Supervision of interns and residents	$ _____	$ _____	$ _____
47. Other (specify)	$ _____	$ _____	$ _____
48.	$ _____	$ _____	$ _____
49. NYC custodian	$ _____	$ _____	$ _____
50. Replacement of equipment	$ _____	$ _____	$ _____
51. Depreciation of buildings	$ _____	$ _____	$ _____
52. Depreciation of equipment	$ _____	$ _____	$ _____

Table 1B–5
Report for Year Ended December 31, 1964: Inpatient Statistical Data

Data	Adults and Children (Col. 1)	Premature Infants (Col. 2)	Newborn Infants (Col. 3)
Accommodation data			
Discharges			
1. Private	_____	_____	_____
2. Semiprivate	_____	_____	_____
3. Ward	_____	_____	_____
4. Total	_____	_____	_____
Patient days			
5. Private	_____	_____	_____
6. Semiprivate	_____	_____	_____
7. Ward	_____	_____	_____
8. Total	_____	_____	_____
Financial status data			
Discharges			
9. Pay or part pay	_____	_____	_____
10. Public charges	_____	_____	_____
11. Free patients	_____	_____	_____
12. Total	_____	_____	_____
Patient days			
13. Pay or part pay	_____	_____	_____
14. Public charges	_____	_____	_____
15. Free patients	_____	_____	_____
16. Total	_____	_____	_____
Miscellaneous			
17. Number of deaths included in discharges	_____	_____	_____
18. Census on last day of year	_____	_____	_____

Class of Service data	Discharges	Patient Days
Adults and children:		
19. Medical-surgical	_____	_____
20. Pediatrics	_____	_____
21. Obstetrics	_____	_____
22. Psychiatric	_____	_____
23. Other (specify)	_____	_____
24. Total	_____	_____

Bed complement	Private	Semiprivate	Ward (Four Beds or Less)	Ward (More Than Four Beds)	All
Adults and children					
25. Medical-surgical	_____	_____	_____	_____	_____
26. Pediatrics	_____	_____	_____	_____	_____
27. Obstetrics	_____	_____	_____	_____	_____
28. Psychiatric	_____	_____	_____	_____	_____
29. Intensive care unit	_____	_____	_____	_____	_____
30.	_____	_____	_____	_____	_____
31. Total	_____	_____	_____	_____	_____
32. Occupancy, % (4)	_____	_____	_____	_____	_____
Newborn bassinets					
33. Premature infants					_____
34. Newborn infants					_____
35. Total					_____

Table 1B–6
Report for Year Ended December 31, 1964: Miscellaneous Statistical Data

Hospital Personnel	Full-Time	Part-Time Number of Employees	Part-Time Weekly Hours Worked
1. Administrative and general			
2. Operation and maintenance of plant			
3. Housekeeping			
4. Laundry and sewing room			
5. Dietary			
6. Clinicians and medical chiefs			
7. Interns and residents			
8. Registered nurses			
9. Licensed practical nurses			
10. Orderlies, aides, and attendants			
11. Student nurses			
12. Social service			
13. Medical records			
14. Pharmacy			
15. Central supply			
16. Operating and recovery rooms			
17. Anesthesia			
18. Delivery rooms			
19. Radiology, diagnostic			
20. Radiology, therapeutic			
21. Laboratory			
22. Electrocardiograph			
23. Physical therapy			
24. Oxygen therapy			
25. Home care treatment			
26. Blood bank			
27. Ambulance			
28. Outpatient clinics			
29. Emergency service			
30. All other employees			
31. Total Employees			

Outpatient Statistics	Number of Visits	Number of Different Individuals
38. Clinic		
39. Emergency department		
40. Private ambulatory patients		

The definition of group 2 hospitals is

> Accredited voluntary general hospitals not included in group 1, rendering at least 125,000 patient days annually (exclusive of newborn days) that meet the following requirements:

1. Full-time physicians serving as residents under an American Medical Association approved residency training program covering at least eight different specialties of which five are clinical specialties which include internal medicine and surgery.
2. A professional nursing school or an affiliation which requires the regular training of professional nursing students on at least two clinical services under an agreement with a college or university offering a degree course in nursing, or, in the absence of the above, full-time physicians serving as interns under an AMA approved internship program.
3. A licensed outpatient department and an emergency service.[4]

All the sample hospitals are voluntary and non-Catholic. Catholic hospitals were excluded because of their use of members of religious

Table 1B–7
Characteristics of Sample Hospitals

	Mean	Standard Deviation	Maximum	Minimum
1961				
Beds	158.66	95.850	417	24
Discharges	5445.1	3343.4	14,065	808
Flow rate	35.332	9.942	61.304	19.763
Ambulatory visits per case	2.833	2.264	11.72	0.0
House staff per case	72.5×10^{-5}	11.7×10^{-4}	31.5×10^{-4}	0.0
Nurse students per case	17.9×10^{-4}	36.9×10^{-4}	16.1×10^{-3}	0.0
Labor cost per case[a]	$189.41	$53.01	$370.20	$92.35
Nonlabor cost per case	$ 97.58	$24.34	$167.62	$50.80
1964				
Beds	169.88	98.959	452	25
Discharges	5919.3	3621.4	14,310	925
Flow rate	34.651	8.024	61.416	16.228
Ambulatory visits per case	3.141	2.305	11.89	0.218
House staff per case	78.0×10^{-5}	13.2×10^{-4}	64.9×10^{-4}	0.0
Nurse students per case	16.6×10^{-4}	33.2×10^{-4}	13.5×10^{-3}	0.0
Labor cost per case[b]	$257.10	$65.97	$490.63	$148.21
Nonlabor cost per case	$118.97	$29.99	$219.74	$ 76.87

[a]Adjusted for wage-rate differences in a manner similar to that described for 1964.
[b]Adjusted for wage-rate differences.

orders whose salary clearly does not reflect the value of their services. With the exception of one local government hospital, all the hospitals are privately owned and operated.

The appropriate definition of cost for the purposes of this study should include only costs attributable to producing the outputs described in the second section of this chapter. The actual definition of cost used here differs from this definition in several respects and for several reasons.

First, depreciation was not included primarily because the depreciation figures are of doubtful validity and because methods of calculating depreciation may differ from hospital to hospital.

Second, only direct expenses that were clearly unrelated to the production of the outputs under consideration could be excluded, since any method of allocating indirect expenses to unrelated activities would be clearly arbitrary. In terms of the 1961 Financial and Statistical Reports (table 1B–1), the excluded expense categories were: 39, 40, 42–46, 48–52. The category "extraordinary repairs and maintenance" was excluded because expenses in this category may reasonably be regarded as capital rather than current expenditures.

Finally, calendar-year expenses are not identical to calendar-year costs to the extent that cost accruals do not correspond to actual payments.

In 1961 three hospitals reported nursing school expense but listed no nursing students in their personnel reports. The number of student nurses in these hospitals was therefore estimated from the following regression.

Number of student nurses =
$$-2.430 + 0.934 \times 10^{-3} \text{ nursing school expense}$$
$$(0.18) \quad (5.22)$$

The coefficients were estimated by OLS; t-values are in parentheses; R^2 was 0.68.

In 1964 one hospital reported nursing school expense but no student nurses. The number of student nurses in this hospital was estimated from the following regression.

Number of student nurses =
$$-8.369 + 0.847 \times 10^{-3} \text{ nursing school expense}$$
$$(0.89) \quad (7.77)$$

This equation also employed OLS; R^2 was 0.78.

Before estimating the average labor cost regressions for 1964, total labor cost for each hospital was deflated by an area wage index and then

Table 1B–8
Average Salaries by Area

Area	Average Annual Salary, 1964
Nassau County	$4,071
Suffolk County	3,929
Orange and Rockland Counties	3,948
Ulster, Sullivan, and Greene Counties	3,628
Columbia, Dutchess, and Putnam Counties	3,665
Westchester County	4,250
New York City	4,298
Delaware County	3,161

multiplied by the index value for the New York City area. The area wage index was computed by first selecting all the sample hospitals in the area that reported personnel in categories 1, 2, and 5 of table 1B–6, the Financial and Statistical Reports for 1964.[5] The total number of full-time-equivalent personnel for each category in each hospital was computed on the assumption that each full-time employee worked forty hours per week. The relevant labor expense figures were then used to compute average yearly salaries for each hospital for each category, and the un-weighted mean salary for each category was then computed for each area.[6]

To determine the weights to give to the mean salary for each category, ten hospitals were selected at random from the total sample and their personnel reports were used to compute the ratio of full-time-equivalent personnel in all the included categories to total full-time-equivalent personnel. The same hospitals were used to compute the ratio of personnel in each category to total personnel, and the weight assigned to each category was this ratio divided by the ratio of all included personnel to total personnel. The weighted average of the mean salaries in the relevant categories was then computed for each area. (The results of these computations are given in table 1B–8.) This weighted average was then divided into total labor cost for each hospital in the area, and the result was multiplied by the weighted average for the New York City area.

Notes

1. The data on medical education were taken from the *Directory of Approved Residencies and Internships*.
2. While tables 1B–1 through 1B–6 are not from one of the sample

hospitals, some data items have been blanked out to preserve the confidentiality of the information contained in the reports.

3. "Proposed Revision of Member Hospital Reimbursement Formula," mimeographed (Associated Hospital Service of New York, 1967), pp. 21–23. Reprinted with permission.

4. Ibid.

5. For the New York City area, rather than include all the hospitals, six hospitals were selected at random.

6. The relevant figures from table 1B–4 are given in lines 1, 2, 4, 8, and 9.

A Microeconometric Study of Hospital Cost Inflation

Hospital costs have been rising rapidly for a long time.[1] And the continuation of this rapid rise into the near future seems certain. This does not mean, however, that the problem of rapidly rising hospital costs should be considered insoluble. The failure to develop a generally effective policy for controlling costs should not be taken as an indication that the cost-inflation process is inevitable or immutable.[2] Rather it is a reflection of ignorance about the process of hospital cost inflation.

The formulation of effective inflation-control policy requires the identification of the causes of cost inflation and information about the quantitative importance of various causes. The analysis described in this chapter attempts to provide some of this information. In particular, it attempts to explain why the rate of cost inflation varies across hospitals and over time and to determine the most important causes of cost inflation.[3]

A behavioral model of hospital cost inflation is presented in the first section. This model is used to develop a relationship between average cost per patient-day in an individual hospital and exogenous variables that influence the hospital's behavior. The second section identifies the variables used in this analysis and describes the data used to estimate the average-cost relationship. The third section presents two types of empirical results: estimated average-cost equations and estimates of the inflationary impact of particular exogenous variables. A further discussion and summary of these results is presented in the fourth section, along with a brief evaluation of the micro approach used in this study.

A Behavioral Model of Hospital Cost Inflation

Most statistical studies of interhospital variations in average cost have used cross-sectional data to estimate relationships between average cost and variables such as size, occupancy rate, and diagnostic mix. These estimated cost functions are probably not very helpful in explaining increases in cost over time, since changes in their independent variables can account for only a small portion of observed inflation.[4] The purpose of this section is to develop an approach to studying interhospital cost variations that will also be useful for studying increases in costs over time.

Let us begin by noting that the demand for the services provided by a particular hospital depends on the price it charges and on a number of other variables that we shall refer to as demand parameters.[5] In mathematical notation

$$Q_{di} = F_d(p_{1i}, D_{1i}, \ldots, D_{ni}) \tag{2.1}$$

where Q_d is quantity demanded (measured in terms of day of care), p is price, and D_j is the jth demand parameter.

The demand function for hospital services F_d is not a demand function in the usual sense. Purchasing hospital care is much more complicated than purchasing household goods. A patient's decision to seek hospital care is typically influenced by his preferences and those of his physician. This decision may also be influenced by the availability of hospital beds and ambulatory services.[6]

Thus while the usual demand function can be derived from the preferences of the purchaser alone, equation 2.1 represents a relationship that emerges from the interaction of the preferences of several individuals and of factors external to those individuals. It is perhaps more accurate to refer to F_d as a price-output function or an output-determination function rather than a demand function. Furthermore, while this discussion assumes that for given values of p_i and the D_{ji}, the quantity of output produced equals Q_{di}, this does not imply that the preferences of any particular individual are satisfied. We shall be guided by tradition, however, and refer to F_d as a demand function.[7]

The terms on which the hospital can purchase factors of production are given by factor-supply functions. To simplify the discussion we assume only one factor N with a supply function:

$$N_{si} = F_s(w_{Ni}, S_{1i}, \ldots, S_{ki}) \tag{2.2}$$

where w_{Ni} is the factor price paid by the ith hospital and S_{ji} is the jth factor-supply parameter.

It is sufficient for our purposes to describe the hospital production relationships as a relationship between the quantity of output Q_i, the quantity of input N_i, a vector of product-mix measures X_i, and a variable that we shall call surplus s_i:

$$Q_i = F_p(N_i, X_i, s_i) \tag{2.3}$$

Surplus may be viewed as an index of "quality" per unit of output, slack costs per unit of output, or both.[8]

The product mix of the hospital X_i is assumed to be determined by p_i and by a group of product-mix parameters $K_{ii}, \ldots, K_{mi}$. That is,

$$X_i = F_x(p_i, K_{ii}, \ldots, K_{mi}) \tag{2.4}$$

The set of relevant product-mix parameters overlaps to a large extent the set of demand parameters. For example, demographic characteristics of the population served by the hospital may affect both the level of demand and the types of cases treated.[9]

Finally, we assume that the decision-making process within the hospital bureaucracy can be described as the maximization of a preference function F_w that contains s_i as one of its arguments.[10] In the most general terms,

$$\mathbf{W}_i = F_w(s_i, M_{1i}, \ldots, M_{vi}, R_{1i}, \ldots, R_{xi}) \tag{2.5}$$

where W_i is the preference index, M_{ji} is the jth maximand (in addition to s_i), and R_{ji} is the jth preference-function parameter.

To maximize W_i the hospital bureaucracy chooses the appropriate optimal values for p_i and N_i. The hospital's optimal output and product mix may then be determined from equations 2.1 and 2.4, and on the assumption that $N_i = N_{si}$, the optimal values for w_{Ni} and for total cost $w_{Ni} \cdot N_i$ may be obtained from equation 2.2. The optimal value of s_i may then be obtained from equation 2.3. Since the choices of P_i and N_i determine the optimal values for output and total cost, they also determine the optimal value for average cost per day, which we shall denote by AC_i^*.

Thus AC_i^* may be considered a function of the parameters previously introduced, that is, the D_{ji}, S_{ji}, K_{ji}, and R_{ji}.[11]

$$AC_i^* = F_c(\ldots, D_{ji}, \ldots, S_{ji}, \ldots, K_{ji}, \ldots, R_{ji}, \ldots) \tag{2.6}$$

And to complete the description of the general model, we add the assumption that the actual average cost in year t in the ith hospital AC_{it} is a function of AC_{it}^*, $AC_{i,t-1}$, and an error term Z_{it}. In particular, we assume a long-proportional adjustment process whereby

$$AC_{it}/AC_{i,t-1} = (AC_{it}^*/AC_{i,t-1})^b \cdot Z_{it} \tag{2.7}$$

where b is the speed-of-adjustment coefficient.[12] Thus by substitution from equation 2.6 and multiplication of $AC_{i,t-1}$, we obtain[13]

$$AC_{it} = [F_c(\ldots, D_{jit}, \ldots, S_{jit}, \ldots, K_{ji}, \ldots, R_{jit}, \ldots)]^b \cdot AC_{i,t-1}^{(1-b)} \cdot Z_{it} \tag{2.8}$$

By specifying a functional form for F_c and estimating the coefficients of equation 2.8, we may determine whether an increase in a particular parameter implies an increase or a decrease in AC_{it}^* and AC_{it}.[14] But without incorporating additional assumptions into the model, it is not possible to predict a priori the effect caused by increases in a particular parameter. Yet it does seem reasonable to expect, for example, that if D_j and D_k $(k \neq j)$ have the same (different) effects on F_d they will also have the same (different) effects on F_c. This will be true if, for example, we assume that

$$Q_{di} = F_{dh}(p_i, H_i), \quad \text{and} \quad H_i = H(D_{1i}, \ldots, D_{ni}) \qquad (2.9)$$

This completes the general description of the behavioral model. This type of model seems more promising than the traditional cost-function model for studying increases in cost over time. Potential causes of hospital cost inflation may affect the level of costs by influencing hospital pricing and input-choice decisions. These potential causes do not, however, appear as explanatory variables in traditional cost functions. Estimation of such a cost function does not permit us to measure the effect of any single potential cause on cost levels.

Within the framework of the behavioral model these potential causes are viewed as parameters and may be included directly in equation 2.8. Estimation of 2.8 thus permits us to determine whether a potential cause has indeed affected the rate of cost inflation and the direction and magnitude of its effect. For example, increases in incomes may have increased the level of costs by increasing the demand for hospital services.[15] To determine whether a relationship exists between income and the level of costs, we simply include income as an explanatory variable in question 2.8.

In the next section I shall make the behavioral model more specific by identifying particular exogenous variables as parameters to be included in the model. I shall also describe the data used for estimating the relationship between AC_{it}, $AC_{i,t-1}$, and these exogenous variables. Results of the estimation process are presented in the third section.[16]

Data and Variables Included in the Analysis

The behavioral model of cost determination will be applied to data from eighty-six nonfederal, nonprofit hospitals in southeastern New York State. (For a description of data sources and adjustments, see appendix 2A.) These hospitals all provide general short-term care and all are community hospitals. That is, none of them is a major teaching or research

Table 2–1
Comparison of Study Hospitals with All Similar U.S. Hospitals

	1961	1962	1963	1964	1965	1966	1967
Average cost per day							
United States	$36.04	$37.77	$39.87	$42.47	$45.40	$48.94	$54.99
New York	$35.47	$37.96	$41.41	$44.11	$47.57	$52.32	$58.60
Percentage increase in average cost per day							
United States		4.80	5.55	6.54	6.89	7.79	12.36
New York		7.02	9.96	6.52	7.84	9.99	12.00
Average length of stay							
United States	7.5	7.6	7.6	7.6	7.7	7.9	8.2
New York	8.3	8.5	8.5	8.6	8.6	9.0	9.4
Occupancy rate							
United States	76.1	76.8	77.7	78.1	77.8	78.5	79.7
New York	76.1	76.3	77.3	77.5	78.0	79.4	82.6
Average bed complement							
United States	121	122	123	126	129	132	135
New York	156	161	166	171	175	177	181

Note: U.S. hospitals are nonfederal short-term general and other special. Data source for these hospitals is [1].

center (even though some do have internship and residency programs). Approximately one-third of these hospitals are located in New York City. Seven cross sections of annual data from these hospitals will be analyzed. The time period excompassed by the data is 1961–1967.[17]

Since the data come from one small geographic area, it is relevant to consider the comparability of the hospitals under study to hospitals across the entire country. The data shown in table 2–1 indicate that the two groups are fairly comparable. The hospitals under study are somewhat larger, have a longer length of stay (defined as total patient-days divided by the total number of cases treated), and have experienced a slightly more rapid pace of cost inflation than similar hospitals throughout the country.

The dependent variable in the regressions reported in the third section is average cost per inpatient-day. Observations on the lagged dependent variable for each hospital run from 1960 to 1966.

The following variables are included as demand parameters.

Population (POP). This variable is intended to measure the number of persons in the market served by the hospital. It is defined as the population of the county in which the hospital is located multiplied by the number of beds in the hospital and divided by the total number of hospital beds in the county.[18] POP is included as a demand parameter because the demand for the series of the ith hospital may be expressed as $POP_i \cdot F_{dpc}(D_{1i}, \ldots, D_{n-1,i})$, where F_{dpc} is the per capita demand function for hospital services. Thus POP should have a positive effect on demand.

Income (INC). This variable is per capita income in the county in which the hospital is located. It is expected to have a positive impact on demand.

Consumer prices (CPI). This variable, the consumer price index for the New York SMSA, is included to reflect changes in the prices of goods and services other than hospital care. Increases in these prices will presumably increase the demand for hospital care by reducing the relative price of such care.

Population density (DEN). This variable is the population density of the county in which the hospital is located. It has been used in studies of the demand for hospital care primarily to reflect the impact of travel distances. There are several reasons for expecting that increases in DEN will decrease the demand for hospital admissions. One is that patients in low-density areas have to travel farther to obtain either hospital care or ambulatory care. Since treatment of a given condition on an ambulatory basis requires several trips to the place where service is provided while inpatient care requires only one, ambulatory treatment becomes less desirable in low-density areas. Similarly, physicians who render care in patients' homes may reduce their own travel time by treating more of their patients in the hospital. Thus physicians in low-density areas may be more likely to recommend hospitalization for their patients.

These reasons would also imply that DEN has a negative effect on average length of stay. On the other hand, as Feldstein has suggested, the impact of density on admission rates may result in a higher proportion of serious cases in high-density areas and hence a longer length of stay.[19]

In addition to these demand parameters, four measures of insurance coverage in the market served by the hospital are included. These measures are the percentage of persons not covered by Blue Cross (BC), the percentage not covered by Medicare (MCARE), the percentage not covered by commercial insurance (COMM), and the percentage not covered by tax-supported welfare programs such as Medicaid (TAX). All these variables presumably have a negative impact on demand because a decrease in any one of them implies an increase in insurance coverage and thus an increase in demand.[20]

It has been argued on several occasions that the appropriate way to include insurance coverage in demand equations is through the use of a net price variable.[21] That is, insurance coverage is represented by some number v between zero and one which, when multiplied by the nominal price, yields the price out-of-pocket price to the patient purchasing care. Since we do not estimate demand directly, however, we do not use a price variable or a net price variable. But we include v directly as the insurance variable.[22]

This approach is rejected (in favor of including the four separate insurance variables just mentioned) for two reasons. First, we are interested in comparing the cost impact of various types of insurance coverage.[23] Second, although we have listed these insurance variables as demand parameters, we do not wish to rule out the possibility that they affect hospital behavior directly (in addition to their effect via increased demand) and that this direct effect varies across types of coverage.

Finally, two measures of physician availability are included as demand parameters.

Non-hospital-based physicians per person (NHMD). This demand parameter is the number of physicians in the county in which the hospital is located divided by county population. The number of physicians includes only those whose major activity was patient care and who were not full-time hospital staff physicians.

GP's and medical specialists per person (GPMS). This demand parameter is the number of general practitioners and medical specialists per person in the county in which the hospital is located. Like NHMD, GPMS does not include full-time hospital staff or physicians not engaged primarily in patient care. Since GPMS includes GPs, internists, and pediatricians, along with some other smaller groupings of specialists, it corresponds very roughly to the notion of primary care physicians.[24]

The availability of physicians of various types may influence the demand for hospital care in several ways. Greater availability of physicians may imply a greater availability of ambulatory care and thus a reduced demand for hospital care.[25] It may also imply relatively smaller patient loads per physician and thus a reduction in the physician's incentive to economize on his own time by hospitalizing a greater percentage of his patients.[26] On the other hand, a greater availability of physicians may increase the demand for hospital care because most patients can be admitted to a hospital only after a physician has evaluated their condition and recommended admission.[27]

Furthermore, availability of certain types of hospital-oriented physicians may have a more positive impact on the demand for hospital care than availability of other types of physicians because the former types tend to treat a larger proportion of their cases on an inpatient basis.[28] Since GPMS is presumed to reflect the availability of primary care physicians who treat many of their patients on an ambulatory basis while NHMD includes *both* primary care physicians and hospital-oriented physicians, NHMD should have a more positive impact on demand than GPMS.

The product mix of the hospital is probably influenced by demand parameters like these. In addition, both demand and product mix are probably affected by demographic characteristics of the population served. To capture the influence of interhospital variation in demographic characteristics, we shall include the variable HSIZE. This is defined as the average household size (in 1960) for the minor civil division (township or borough) in which the hospital is located.[29] Since a large value for HSIZE probably indicates a large proportion of children in the county population, we expect HSIZE to be negatively related to demand.

Two variables have been included as factor-supply parameters.

Service industry wages (SWAGE). SWAGE, the average weekly earnings in the service industries of the county, is included to account for the effect of labor-market conditions on hospital costs. Wages in the service industry should be a better index of labor market conditions confronting a hospital than, say, manufacturing wages because of the importance of low-skill labor in hospitals. An increase in SWAGE will cause an upward (leftward) shift in the horizontal (upward-sloping) labor supply curve of the hospital.

Wholesale prices (WPI). The wholesale price index is included to reflect supply conditions for nonlabor inputs. As with SWAGE, increases in WPI are assumed to imply upward shifts in factor-supply functions.

Two additional variables that have been included cannot be classified simply in terms of the behavioral model. One is an index of urbanization (URB) for the county. URB may be viewed as a preference-function parameter in that isolated rural hospitals may have organizational goals different from those of hospitals in an urban area. URB is also included to correct for intercounty variations in the prices of other goods and services and the prices of nonlabor inputs. CPI and WPI vary only across years. Thus they cannot reflect the effects of such intercounty variations on costs.

The second variable is the number of beds in the hospital (BEDS). For a given value of POP, BEDS indicates the availability of hospital beds for persons in the market served by the hospital. Thus an increase in beds implies an increase in the demand for hospital services.[30]

But BEDS may also be regarded as a preference-function parameter. For example, a hospital with more beds probably wants to supply a greater quantity of services than one with fewer beds. If both hospitals face identical demand conditions, the hospital with more beds must charge a lower price to generate a quantity demanded consistent with its larger desired output. But then its level of average cost must be lower unless its per unit profit (deficit) is sufficiently smaller (larger) than the per unit profit (deficit) of the smaller hospital. The larger hospital presumably offsets some of this reduction in per unit profit by reducing the level of average cost (and probably the level of surplus).

Although the behavioral model outlined in the first section is too general to permit us to rigorously derive hypotheses about the way in which particular variables affect cost levels, it seems reasonable to conjecture that increases in demand and upward shifts in factor-supply functions have positive effects on cost. This implies that the following variables are expected to have positive coefficients in the average-cost equations: POP, INC, CPI, SWAGE, and WPI. Similarly, HSIZE, BC, MCARE, COMM, TAX, and DEN are expected to display negative coefficients. To the extent that URB reflects differences in the prices of inputs as well as goods and services, it should have a positive coefficient. Since the impacts of GPMS and NHMD on demand are not clear, it is difficult to predict the signs of their coefficients although we expect GPMS to have a less positive (or more negative) coefficient than NHMD. Finally, the sign of the coefficient of BEDS depends on the relative magnitudes of its positive impact on cost (through its effect on demand) and its negative impact on cost (through its effect on hospital preferences).

Empirical Results

By assuming a multiplicative form for F_c and by taking logarithms of both sides of equation 2.8, we obtain an equation that is linear in the coefficients to be estimated. This section presents the results obtained by estimating the coefficients of such an equation. The dependent variable is average cost per day in the ith hospital in year t (AC_{it}). The lagged dependent variable ($AC_{i,t-1}$) and the insurance variables are treated as endogenous, and an instrumental-variables procedure is employed.[31]

Table 2–2 presents the results of the estimation process. The most striking aspect of these results is the low estimated values for the speed-of-adjustment coefficient (which is one minus the coefficient of AC_{t-1}). These estimates are all between 0.0796 and 0.0838, indicating that less than one-tenth of the difference in logarithms between AC_{it} and AC_{it}^* is made up within the year.[32]

The coefficients for the insurance variables are highly significant and negative, indicating that an increase in insurance coverage increases average cost per day. It is interesting to compare the relative impact of the different insurance variables since the corresponding forms of coverage differ in several respects. Commercial insurance is primarily of the indemnity-benefit type (paying a fixed sum per day for room and board), with additional reimbursement based on ancillary service charges to the patient. Blue Cross, Medicare, and tax-supported welfare insurance are cost-based plans that provide service benefits. Differences may also exist in the extent to which nonhospital care is covered under the various plans,

Table 2–2
Average-Cost-per-Day Equations
(t-ratios in parentheses)

	Equation				
	2.10	*2.11*	*2.12*	*2.13*	*2.14*
AC_{t-1}	0.9180	0.9177	0.9195	0.9204	0.9182
	(45.29)	(45.42)	(42.33)	(45.64)	(45.54)
POP	0.0288	0.0271	0.0414	0.0342	0.0246
	(1.43)	(1.44)	(2.72)	(1.97)	(1.28)
BEDS	−0.0269	−0.0253	−0.0391	−0.2037	−0.0224
	(1.24)	(1.23)	(2.22)	(1.70)	(1.08)
BC	−0.1306	−0.1284	−0.1323	−0.1349	−0.1262
	(3.37)	(3.52)	(3.55)	(3.61)	(3.22)
COMM	−0.2523	−0.2500	−0.2442	−0.2605	−0.2478
	(3.45)	(3.51)	(3.43)	(3.59)	(3.37)
MCARE	−0.1390	−0.1375	−0.1421	−0.1442	−0.1343
	(2.83)	(2.87)	(2.92)	(2.95)	(2.72)
TAX	−0.2162	−0.2140	−0.2160	−0.2260	−0.2083
	(3.48)	(3.56)	(3.53)	(3.72)	(3.32)
SWAGE	0.0277	0.0259	0.0316	—	0.0427
	(0.81)	(0.77)	(1.07)		(1.62)
INC	−0.0092	—	—	—	−0.0110
	(0.25)				(0.30)
CPI	0.3088	0.2838	0.2680	0.3028	0.3098
	(1.38)	(1.39)	(1.32)	(1.51)	(1.39)
WPI	0.5063	0.5057	0.4968	0.5026	0.5046
	(1.55)	(1.55)	(1.53)	(1.54)	(1.55)
HSIZE	−0.0702	−0.0706	−0.0532	0.0653	−0.0711
	(1.70)	(1.71)	(1.43)	(1.79)	(1.73)
URB	0.303	0.0260	—	0.0135	0.0371
	(1.08)	(1.21)		(1.31)	(1.45)
GPMS	−0.0347	−0.0417	−0.0455	−0.0642	−0.0093
	(0.70)	(1.00)	(1.21)	(1.78)	(0.29)
NHMD	0.0263	0.0276	0.0435	0.0554	—
	(0.67)	(0.71)	(1.30)	(2.05)	
DEN	−0.0043	−0.0033	—	—	−0.0058
	(0.75)	(0.83)			(1.13)
CONSTANT	−0.5969	−0.5227	−0.2033	−0.2334	−0.8116
	(0.30)	(0.26)	(0.10)	(0.12)	(0.41)
$R(AC_t, AC_t^*)$	—	0.687	0.682	0.671	—

Table 2–2 continued

	Equation				
	2.15	2.16	2.17	2.18	2.19
AC_{t-1}	0.9181 (45.64)	0.9185 (45.70)	0.9178 (45.66)	0.9180 (45.65)	0.9162 (46.31)
POP	0.0218 (1.16)	0.0277 (1.45)	0.0224 (1.28)	0.0291 (2.46)	0.0329 (2.91)
BEDS	−0.0199 (0.97)	−0.0253 (1.22)	−0.0202 (1.05)	−0.0269 (1.91)	−0.0316 (2.29)
BC	−0.1205 (3.19)	−0.1192 (3.14)	−0.1232 (3.36)	−0.1286 (3.25)	−0.1243 (3.34)
COMM	−0.2440 (3.36)	−0.2352 (3.29)	−0.2448 (3.42)	−0.2508 (3.38)	−0.2480 (3.40)
MCARE	−0.1320 (2.70)	−0.1311 (2.68)	−0.1323 (2.75)	−0.1359 (2.73)	−0.1330 (2.75)
TAX	−0.2023 (3.30)	−0.1984 (3.25)	−0.2052 (3.40)	−0.2119 (3.33)	−0.2107 (3.35)
SWAGE	0.0411 (1.56)	0.0499 (1.93)	0.0415 (1.59)	0.0424 (1.29)	0.0368 (1.42)
INC	0.0195 (0.82)	0.0225 (0.81)	—	−0.0188 (0.72)	—
CPI	0.2165 (1.02)	0.2002 (0.94)	0.2798 (1.38)	0.3426 (1.84)	0.3229 (1.73)
WPI	0.5057 (1.56)	0.4971 (1.54)	0.5037 (1.55)	0.5017 (1.55)	0.4902 (1.52)
HSIZE	−0.0614 (1.55)	−0.0549 (1.41)	−0.0716 (1.75)	−0.0696 (1.72)	−0.0677 (1.69)
URB	0.0115 (1.02)	—	0.0322 (1.66)	0.0394 (1.60)	0.0278 (1.51)
GPMS	−0.0272 (0.95)	−0.0223 (0.72)	−0.0162 (0.70)	—	—
NHMD	—	—		—	—
DEN	—	0.0009 (0.40)	−0.0047 (1.38)	−0.0066 (1.44)	−0.0044 (1.32)
CONSTANT	−0.4194 (0.21)	−0.3392 (0.17)	−0.7347 (0.37)	−0.8804 (0.45)	−0.7873 (0.40)
$R(AC_t, AC_t^*)$	0.692	—	0.692	—	0.692

Note: All equations are in double-log form. The dependent variable in each equation is the logarithm of average cost per patient-day. The squared correlation between fitted and observed values for AC_t is approximately 0.94 in all equations.

Table 2-3
Ratios of Partial Derivatives for Mean Coverage Levels

Equation	Year	MCARE/BC	COMM/BC	TAX/BC
2.12	1961	—	0.972	0.821
2.12	1967	1.074	1.386	1.201
2.19	1961	—	1.051	0.852
2.19	1967	1.070	1.499	1.247

and these differences may affect the impact of each type of coverage on costs.

The regression results consistently show larger coefficients for COMM and TAX than for BC and MCARE. Thus if all four types of coverage are equally widespread, the elasticity of AC_t and the partial derivative of AC_t with respect to increases in coverage will be larger for COMM and TAX. But the four types of coverage are not, in fact, equally widespread. It is therefore relevant to compare the cost impact of increases in each of the types of coverage in the average hospital. This comparison is drawn in table 2-3, which presents ratios of partial derivatives of AC_t with respect to insurance variables calculated from mean coverage levels in 1961 and in 1967.

Table 2-3 reveals generally small differences in cost impact across types of coverage, although increases in commercial insurance seem to be the most inflationary. This result is surprising given the general consensus that cost-based reimbursement plans are more inflationary than indemnity and charge-based plans.[33] On the other hand, limitations on reimbursable cost levels in Blue Cross[34] and the threat (if not the reality) of cost and utilization review under Medicare may serve to dampen the inflationary impact of these types of coverage. Payment delays and the resulting cash-flow problems in welfare insurance programs may lead to the same result. Also commercial insurance may provide the narrowest coverage for nonhospital services, and this may explain the finding.[35]

One should not make too much of this, however. The evidence that commercial insurance has a greater inflationary impact is hardly overwhelming. But the results are surprising in that they do not support the notion that cost-based plans are more inflationary.

The negative coefficients for the insurance variables are consistent with the conjecture that increases in demand have a positive impact on cost. The positive coefficients for POP and CPI, which are almost always larger than their standard errors, are also consistent with this conclusion.[36]

In general, INC seems to have no clear impact on cost levels. While this result is not inconsistent with the findings of other investigators,[37] it is surprising in view of conclusions derived from the traditional theory of consumer behavior. That is, we would not expect hospital care to be on the borderline between an inferior and a normal good.

There are at least two reasons why increases in income may not have a clear, positive impact on the demand for hospital care. The first is that increases in income may be positively related to improvements in health status and to the increased use of preventive rather than acute medical care. The second is that the process of consuming hospital care requires substantial amounts of time on the part of the consumers. As income increases, the value of the time-cost of hospital care increases, thus reducing demand.[38]

A larger value for HSIZE is presumably associated with a greater proportion of children in the population. Thus we expect that both the case-mix effects and the demand effects of HSIZE result in a negative impact on cost. This expectation is consistent with the finding that the coefficient of HSIZE is consistently negative and substantially larger than its standard error.

The negative and generally significant coefficients for BEDS indicate that, in terms of their effects on cost, the increase in demand due to increased bed availability is outweighed by the change in the hospital's preferences regarding optimal output levels resulting from an increase in BEDS. Furthermore, these coefficients are almost exactly equal in absolute value to the coefficients of POP. This suggests that the results would be basically unchanged if POP and BEDS were replaced by the single variable POP/BEDS (or BEDS/POP).[39]

The signs of the coefficients for SWAGE and WPI confirm the expectation that upward shifts in factor-supply functions lead to cost increases. These coefficients (especially those for WPI) are in most cases clearly larger than their standard errors.[40]

Although the estimated coefficients of the physician availability variables do not exceed their standard errors in a number of instances, the fact that NHMD has a more positive impact on cost is consistent with a priori expectations (given the positive association between demand and cost). In equations 2.10–2.13 the negative coefficients for GPMS are larger in absolute value than the positive coefficients for NHMD. Since GPMS is always less than NHMD, the results indicate that additional GPs and medical specialists per capita will actually lower cost levels.

Finally, the results for DEN and URB are consistent with our previous findings regarding cost responses to demand and factor-supply shifts. That is, URB is presumed to be positively associated with factor-price and consumer-price differences while DEN is presumed to be negatively associated with demand. Positive coefficients for URB and negative coefficients for DEN are in accordance with these presumptions.

The equations in table 2–2 also suggest the presence of some collinearity problems. When URB, DEN, GPMS, NHMD, and SWAGE are all included, as in equation 2.10, the t-values for their coefficients are fairly low. Furthermore, when one or several of these variables are excluded, the absolute size and t-value for the coefficients of the remaining included variables in this set generally increase by substantial amounts.[41] This collinearity allows only tentative conclusions about the magnitude and significance of the effect any one of these variables has on cost.

Observations on all five of these variables are drawn from the county in which the hospital is located. The less-than-satisfactory results for these variables are probably related to the general problem that the county is too large a unit of observation.[42]

Since the data are pooled and a dependent variable is included, it is not very surprising that the R^2's obtained are quite high. A more stringent test of the model's explanatory power is provided by the correlation between the values for AC_{it}^* derived from a particular equation and the value for AC_{it}.[43] This correlation coefficient (denoted by $R(AC_t, AC_t^*)$ in table 2–2) is between 0.65 and 0.70. Given that the model is applied to micro data, these values for $R(AC_t, AC_t^*)$ are surprisingly high.

We shall now turn to the problem of measuring the inflationary impact of particular variables and groups of variables over the 1961–1967 period. This impact could be expressed in terms of rates of increase of actual cost or equilibrium cost.[44] For example, to calculate the impact of changes in TAX on increases in AC_t^*, we simply compare the mean values for AC_{67}^*/AC_{61}^* and $\overline{AC_{67}^*}/AC_{61}^*$. We define $\overline{AC_{67}^*} = AC_{67}^* \cdot (TAX_{61}/TAX_{67})^h$, where h is the elasticity of AC_t^* with respect to TAX, calculated from the estimated coefficients of TAX and AC_{t-1}. The difference between these mean values is the estimated impact of TAX on the rate of increase in AC_t^*. An analogous (but slightly more complex) procedure is employed to calculate the impact on inflation in AC_t.[45]

The results of these calculations should be interpreted cautiously. First, the explanatory variables might not be exogenous. Second, even if they are independent of error terms in the cost-determination equation, they may still depend on the average level of cost (or the average rate of cost inflation) for all hospitals in the sample. Third, some of these variables may be sensitive to changes in other explanatory variables. For example, increases in income may lead to increases in physician availability so that an accurate estimate of the inflationary impact of changes in income would require calculation of direct cost effects and indirect effects (operating through changes in physician availability).

Table 2–4
Contribution to Increases in AC_t and AC^*_t, 1961–1967

Equation Percentage Increase in Contribution of	2.12 $AC^*_t = 188.6$	2.12 $AC_t = 65.4$	2.19 $AC^*_t = 179.7$	2.19 $AC_t = 65.4$
MCARE	151.9	13.6	137.7	12.7
All insurance variables	36.2	4.4	29.9	4.3
GPMS, NHMD	20.1	2.9	—	—
SWAGE	25.9	3.8	28.1	4.3
CPI	98.8	15.0	108.3	17.8
WPI	84.0	10.2	78.4	10.0
Demand variables[a]	133.8	21.1	125.4	21.1
Factor-supply variables[b]	102.4	13.7	98.6	14.1
All variables	188.6	33.1	179.7	33.4

[a]Demand variables include POP, BEDS, DEN, CPI, MCARE, BC, TAX, COMM, GPMS, and NHMD.
[b]Factor-supply variables are WPI and SWAGE.

In conclusion, this method for attributing cost increases to particular factors may lead us astray if these criticisms are applicable. These criticisms may also apply to the use of this method for cost prediction. With these caveats in mind, we shall now turn to the results presented in table 2–4.

Over the 1961–1967 period MCARE, CPI, and WPI all accounted separately for substantial increases in AC^*_t. For example, using equation 2.12 we estimate that if all other explanatory variables had assumed their actual values in 1967 while MCARE had assumed its 1961 value, the increase in AC_t over the 1961–1967 period would have only been 51.8 percent (65.4 percent minus 13.6 percent). Since the advent of Medicare obviously caused a reduction in other types of coverage, it is also relevant to consider the combined impact of all insurance variables. The impact of these variables taken together is only about one-third of the impact of Medicare.[46]

I have also compared the simultaneous impact of all demand variables and the impact of all factor-supply variables. As is indicated in table 2–4, the impact of the demand variables is somewhat larger.[47]

Further Discussion of Results and Concluding Remarks

The empirical analysis has revealed that the actual level of average cost responds quite slowly to changes in the equilibrium level of cost. This response lag may be due to uncertainty or to lack of knowledge on the part of the hospital bureaucracy with regard to its own operations and the market conditions in which it operates. It may also reflect institutional constraints on the hospital's behavior. If these constraints significantly affect the course of cost inflation, further work on identifying the exact nature of these constraints will be an important input to inflation-control policy.[48]

The existence of this lag has important implications for the task of evaluating reimbursement mechanisms and their ability to control costs. Several studies have attempted to compare cost-based reimbursement schemes with charge-based schemes and to isolate the additional impact on cost levels of cost-based schemes.[49] These studies have relied primarily on cross-sectional analyses and have used nondynamic cost functions. My findings, however, indicate that present cost levels are strongly influenced by past conditions and that inclusion of a lagged dependent variable (or use of some other dynamic specification) is necessary to account for the effects of these past conditions.[50]

I have estimated that the size of the cost-response lag is substantial. This finding has rather pessimistic implications for policy. It implies that the recent increases in inflation rates will be slow to disappear even if no important new inflationary forces come into play in the near future. For example, my results indicate an increase of about 180 percent in equilibrium cost over the 1961–1969 period. Since actual cost increased by only 65.4 percent, a continued high rate of inflation is to be expected unless a strong inflation-control policy is put into effect.[51]

My results also indicate that inflation outside the hospital sector, as measured by increases in CPI and WPI, has a very large impact on the rate of cost increase. The estimated coefficients of CPI and WPI are surprisingly large, however, indicating perhaps that this result was in part based on omission of other upward-trending variables.[52]

An alternative but related explanation of this result is that the external institutional forces that serve to restrain the rate of cost increase may be affected directly by increases in CPI or WPI. It seems reasonable to expect that these forces can impose a smaller degree of restraint when inflation outside the hospital sector is intense. The scenario might begin with the local Blue Cross company's citing the rapid general inflation in its application to the state insurance commissioner for a rate increase. The Blue Cross company in turn might look more favorably on given cost increases in individual hospitals and so on. Since this shift in external institutional forces is not measured or included in these regressions, the resulting estimates of the coefficient for CPI and WPI reflect the impact of this shift as well as the direct effects of CPI and WPI.

The calculations of inflationary impact (table 2–4) indicate that both demand and factor-supply variables have been important contributors to recent cost inflation, although the demand variables have been somewhat more important. Furthermore, my estimates imply that the impact of insurance on inflation has not been as large as has been suggested elsewhere.[53]

Finally, my results concerning the negative cost impact of additional hospital beds are similar to those obtained elsewhere.[54]

While these conclusions are clearly supported by the empirical results, the exploratory nature of this analysis suggests that they should be regarded as tentative. There are several areas in which further development of this micro model would be desirable. First, the data are from counties, but the county may be too large a geographical unit to accurately depict the market conditions facing the individual hospital. Similarly, the estimates of the impact of insurance coverage would be improved by better data in this area. Second, the measurement of the total impact of exogenous parameters could be improved by making the number of beds in the hospital an endogenous variable and by estimating the impact of these exogenous parameters on bed supply. Third, better information on factor-supply parameters is needed. Additional parameters relevant to the determination of wage levels for nurses and other technically trained personnel should be added.

More fundamentally, should further effort be devoted to micro models of this type? Or should attention be directed to refining more aggregative approaches to the cost-inflation problem? I shall try to suggest why further work at the micro level seems warranted.

First, a number of important issues are related to the comparative performance of institutions with different characteristics (profit versus nonprofit, public versus private). At an aggregate level it is difficult to confront these issues, since there may be little interstate variation in the preponderance of hospitals of a particular type. Observations on individual units or small geographic areas are necessary. Second, micro models can be used to study the effect on costs of various reimbursement experiments. If these experiments involve geographic areas substantially smaller than a state, it is difficult to measure their effectiveness in a model that is based on data aggregated to the state level. But a micro model could be used effectively to estimate a cost prediction model and determine whether hospitals in the experiment experienced lower-than-predicted costs. Even if the experiment involved an entire state, a micro model would probably still be more effective than an aggregate model in studying the experiment's effects.

The development of and experimentation with new reimbursement methods offers a promising area for development of cost-control policies and for application of a micro model. But the potential of micro studies in this area will not be realized unless the designers of such experiments make provision for the necessary data at the local level.

Notes

1. Unless otherwise noted, the term *hospital costs, hospital cost*, and *cost* refer to average cost per patient-day.

2. Even though it may be possible to control hospital cost inflation, it has been argued that such control might not be desirable. In particular, Anderson and Neuhauser [4] argue that controlling inflation, stifles technological progress in the health industry. Interesting discussions of the case for controlling cost inflation are presented by Evans [12, chap. 1] and M. Feldstein [15, sec. 6]. Klarman presents a thorough consideration of specific ways in which total health care costs might be controlled [18, 21].

3. As M. Feldstein has noted [14], increases in employment and wages and decreases (or lack of increases) in average labor productivity within the hospital industry are primarily the results and not the causes of the inflationary process. Previous studies that focused on these changes have indicated more about how costs have increased than about why they have increased. A few recent studies [14, 22], have applied econometric techniques to analyze the reasons for cost inflation.

4. In other words, if cost inflation is decomposed into the effects of changes in independent variables in a traditional cost function and the effects of changes in the coefficients of that function, the latter effects are probably more important. For an example of how traditional cost functions can be used to study cost inflation, see Salkever [30, chaps. 1, 2]. The major result obtained in that study, that product-mix change accounts for only a small fraction of observed inflation, supports the view that the usefulness of these cost functions in studying cost behavior over time is limited.

5. Variables included in the model that are assumed to be outside the direct control of the hospital bureaucracy are referred to as *parameters*.

6. Notice also that F_d is the demand function for hospital days and might also be written as $\text{ADM}_d(\ ) \cdot \text{MS}_d(\ )$, where ADM_d is the demand function for hospital admissions and MS_d is the functional relationship determining average length of stay. The most thorough discussion of the concept of demand for medical services has been provided by P. Feldstein [16]. The effect of availability on demand is discussed in detail in [14, 15, and 28].

7. This type of demand function has been employed in a number of other studies of the hospital industry. See, for example, [11 and 14].

8. Slack costs are excess costs incurred because the management of the hospital is unwilling to undertake all the cost-cutting and efficiency programs that would be necessary to reduce the cost of producing a given output to the technologically determined minimum. For a further discus-

sion of this, see Evans [12, chap. 2]. If s_i is an indicator of quality (however defined), it could reasonably be included as an argument of F_d, but its inclusion would not alter the form of the cost relationship presented in equation 2.8.

Finally, Q_i could easily be replaced by admissions and mean stay. Denoting these by Q_{Ai} and Q_{si} respectively, we would then write $F_p(N_i, Q_{Ai}, Q_{si}, Z_i, s_i) = 0$.

9. The inclusion of a product-mix determination equation is based on the assumption that the demands for care of different diagnoses may be changed in a nonproportionate fashion by changes in price or in one of the K_{ji}'s. Results presented by M. Feldstein [13, chap. 7] and by Rafferty [26] support this assumption.

10. The assumption that quality or slack costs are viewed by the hospital as desirable has been incorporated in a number of formal models of hospital decision making [12, 14, 24]. A model that does not incorporate this assumption is presented in [8].

11. The existence of this functional relationship depends on the characteristics of the functions F_d, F_p, F_s, and F_w. My purposes here, however, are simply to suggest the theoretic basis for a relationship between AC_i^* and the various parameters and (in the third and fourth sections) to test for the existence of this relationship. Since we are not interested in testing the implications of a particular decision-making model (such as those outlined in [8, 14, and 24]), we shall simply assume that F_c exists.

12. Possible reasons for the existence of a lagged rather than instantaneous adjustment process are discussed in the fourth section.

13. It is clear that incorporation into the analysis of the changes mentioned in notes 6 and 8 would not alter the general form of equation 2.8.

14. For obvious reasons, we shall assume a multiplicative form for F_c.

15. M. Feldstein [15] discusses in detail the effect of increasing demand on cost levels.

16. These results do not constitute a test of the model just outlined, however, because of the model's generality. In other words, the model should be viewed as a heuristic device. It serves to indicate the rationale for including different types of variables in the regression analysis; it does not logically imply the inclusion of specific variables.

17. Hospitals classified as either group 1 or group 2 by the Associated Hospital Service of New York were excluded from the study. These excluded hospitals were so classified because they met the following requirements: (1) rendered at least 125,000 patient-days of care, (2) offered at least eight AMA-approved residency training programs, (3) of-

fered a professional nurse training program or AMA-approved internship program, and (4) operated an outpatient department and an emergency service. For further details see [5].

18. This definition of the number of persons in the market served by the hospital is also used in [9].

19. M. Feldstein's results [14] indicate that density has a significantly positive impact on average length of stay.

20. These variables are defined as the percentage *not* covered to avoid the problem caused by taking logarithms of a variable that takes a value of zero for some observations.

Data on BC, MCARE, COM, and TAX are drawn from inpatient censuses conducted in the sample hospitals in 1961, 1964, and 1967. Observations for other years were obtained by interpolation and extrapolation (see the appendix to this chapter). Thus the data may be inaccurate as measures of coverage in the market served by the hospital. Since this implies measurement error, and since the percentage of inpatients with a particular kind of coverage may depend on the hospital's price (and thus on average cost), these insurance variables are treated as endogenous for estimation purposes.

21. See [14] and [16].

22. This procedure is used in [14].

23. If v is used as the only insurance variable, we are in effect assuming that the difference in cost impacts between types of coverage is determined by the differences in the impact on v of increases in each type of coverage.

24. The specialties included in GPMS, according to [3], are general practice, allergy, cardiovascular diseases, dermatology, gastroenterology, internal medicine, pediatrics, pediatric allergy, pediatric cardiology, pulmonary disease. Those included in NHMD but not in GPMS are general surgery, neurological surgery, obstetrics and gynecology, ophthalmology, orthopedic surgery, otolaryngology, plastic surgery, colon and rectal surgery, thoracic surgery, urology, aviation medicine, anesthesiology, child psychiatry, diagnostic radiology, forensic pathology, neurology, occupational medicine, psychiatry, pathology, physical medicine and rehabilitation, general preventive medicine, public health, radiology, therapeutic radiology.

25. M. Feldstein discusses the rationale for using availability in demand equations in detail. See [14].

26. This point is made by Paul Feldstein [16].

27. The role of the physician as gatekeeper to the hospital has been discussed in [21] and [28]. If there is excess demand for physician services, the fact that physicians play such a role implies that increased physician availability may increase the demand for hospital services.

28. M. Feldstein [14] distinguishes between GPs and hospital-oriented specialists.

29. Other demographic variables were included in preliminary analyses. When these other variables were included with HSIZE, their estimated coefficients were always clearly insignificant, and they were therefore dropped from the analysis. This probably indicates that HSIZE is highly correlated with a variety of demographic characteristics.

30. While measures of physician availability (GPMS and NHMD) and a measure of hospital bed availability (BEDS) are included, the meaning of *availability* may not be the same in these two cases. A measure of availability can be included in a demand function to account for non-monetary price variables such as waiting time. But it may also serve as a supply proxy in a market where excess demand is present and supply determines the level of output. It has been suggested [14] that the former interpretation is correct for measures of the availability of hospital beds while the latter interpretation is correct for measures of physician availability.

31. Instruments were obtained by a ranking procedure similar to that described in [13, pp. 80–81].

32. M. Feldstein [14] obtained estimated adjustment speeds that were higher than those reported here but still quite slow. His results indicated adjustment speeds on the order of 25 percent.

33. Klarman [20] discusses the possible effects of reliance on cost-based plans. A study of average cost per case in a similar group of hospitals [30, chap. 3] found that Medicare coverage in particular had a significant cost impact while other types of coverage did not. But the impact of age on length of stay could explain this result. More generally, the results of that study regarding insurance coverage should be viewed with suspicion for a number of reasons. Only one cross section of data was employed, all explanatory variables were treated as exogenous (including the lagged dependent variable), and several important variables were omitted. Thus the fact that these results are not consistent with the present findings is not a cause for concern.

34. For a description of the limitations applicable to the same hospitals see [7, p. 45].

35. Davis and Russell [11] studied the demands for outpatient care and hospital care and found that Blue Cross coverage and commercial coverage affected these demands differently. Their findings are consistent with the fact that commercial insurance provides less out-of-hospital coverage than Blue Cross.

36. Since these coefficients are estimated by instrumental variables, we cannot apply the significance tests used for OLS coefficients. In view of the asymptomatic normality of the estimated coefficients, however,

and the fact that there are 602 observations in the sample, we should note that t-statistics of 1.289 or larger with only 120 degrees of freedom are 90 percent significant in one-tailed tests.

37. For example, M. Feldstein [14] found that while income had a significantly positive effect on average length of stay, its effect on admissions was clearly insignificant. Russell's cross-sectional studies of hospital admissions and length of stay for both the Medicare and non-Medicare populations revealed either no significant impact of income or a significantly negative impact [28].

38. Holtmann [17] provides an interesting discussion of time costs and behavior of the consumer of medical services.

39. In other words, very similar results would have been obtained if the entire model had been reformulated in per capita terms. This empirical result is consistent with the a priori assumptions of constant returns to scale, horizontal factor-supply curves, and a hospital preference function that includes the occupancy rate rather than total output as an argument. A model embodying these assumptions is presented in [14].

40. The estimated coefficients for WPI and for CPI are suspiciously large. This point is discussed further in the fourth section.

41. This is also somewhat true for the coefficients of POP and BEDS.

42. The counties in the study are highly urbanized or large in area. Thus there are on average more than five hospitals per county.

43. This test has been suggested and applied by M. Feldstein [14].

44. The former approach has previously been used by Salkever [30], while Feldstein employed the latter approach [14].

45. To calculate the impact of increases in, say, TAX on AC_t, we first calculate the impact on AC_t from 1961 to 1962. This generates an adjusted value for AC_{t-1} which is used in predicting AC_t in 1963 and so on. The results thus depend on the time path of change in a variable throughout the 1961–1967 period.

46. From 1965 to 1967 the mean value for Medicare coverage increased from 0 percent to 34.4 percent, while the mean value for the sum of all insurance coverage measures increased by only 10.0 percentage points (from 82.7 percent to 92.7 percent).

47. The demand variables correspond to the variables included in demand functions such as those estimated by Feldstein [14].

48. Lave and Lave [22] suggest that these constraints may depend on "pressure from Blue Cross, patients, and conscientious doctors." (p. 382)

49. See [10] and [25].

50. Klarman [19] has expressed a similar criticism of this type of cross-sectional study.

51. Notice that we have estimated what might be regarded as a short-run model for determining AC_t^*. That is, an increase in, say, CPI

might lead to a long-run impact on AC_t^* smaller than the estimated impact because of a response in bed-supply levels as well as cost levels. To the extent that this long-run response is smaller, these pessimistic conclusions (based on a slow cost-response speed and a large discrepancy between percentage increases in AC_t and AC_t^*) should be moderated.

52. Several regressions were run with a time-trend variable. The estimated coefficient of this variable was negative, and its inclusion increased slightly the magnitude of the coefficients for CPI and WPI.

53. Feldstein [14] obtains a large estimated impact for insurance when he constrains the coefficient of his insurance variable to be equal to the coefficient of the price variable in his demand equations; but when this constraint is dropped, the resulting estimate for the impact of insurance becomes similar to those estimates reported here.

54. See [14].

Appendix 2A
Data Sources and
Adjustments

COMM, TAX, MCARE, BC. These variables are derived from data on primary source of payment obtained in one-day inpatient censuses conducted in 1961, 1964, and 1967 (for further information, see [6].) Data for 1962 and 1963 were obtained by simple interpolation of the 1961 and 1964 data. Since the pattern of insurance coverage changed substantially with the advent of Medicare and Medicaid in 1966, data for 1965 were obtained by simple extrapolation of 1961 and 1964 data. Data for 1966 were calculated as the average of 1967 observations and extrapolations from 1961 to 1965. (A simple average was used since Medicare began on July 1, 1966, and Medicaid on May 1, 1966, in New York State.)

GPMS, NHMD. Observations for the years 1963–1967 were obtained from [2] and [3]. Data for 1961 and 1962 were obtained by simple extrapolation of 1963 and 1965 data on the numbers of physicians and by dividing these numbers by the 1961 and 1962 population figures.

AC_t, AC, AC_{t-1}. These variables were obtained from hospital cost records of the Associated Hospital Service of New York. For a complete description of these records and the cost measures employed, see [30, appendix to chap. 2].

Data on beds in the hospital and in the short-term general hospitals of the county in which it is located were obtained from [1]. Data on county population and INC were taken from [29]. Figures on county area and URB were taken from [31], while data on SWAGE and HSIZE were obtained from [23] and [32] respectively. Finally, data on CPI and WPI are given in [33].

References

1. American Hospital Association. *Hospitals, Journal of the American Hospital Association*, Guide Issues, annual.

2. American Medical Association. *Distribution of Physicians in the U.S.*, annual, 1963–1965.

3. ———. *Distribution of Physicians, Hospitals, and Hospital Beds in the U.S.*, annual since 1966.

4. Anderson, Odin W., and Neuhauser, Duncan. "Rising Costs Are

Inherent in Modern Health Care Systems." *Hospitals, Journal of the American Hospital Association,* February 16, 1969.

5. Associated Hospital Service of New York. "Member Hospital Reinbursement Formula: Effective January 1, 1970," mimeographed.

6. ———. "Hospital Service in Southern New York," mimeographed.

7. ———. *Member Hospital Reimbursement Formula: Review Committee Decisions and Administrative Interpretations Through December 31, 1965.* New York, 1966.

8. Davis, Karen. "A Theory of Economic Behavior in Non-Profit Private Hospitals." Ph.D. dissertation, Rice University, 1969.

9. ———. "Production and Cost Function Estimation for Non-Profit Hospitals," Rice University, 1970.

10. ———. "The Impact of Cost Reimbursement Schemes on Hospital Costs," Social Security Administration, 1971.

11. Davis, Karen, and Russell, Louise B. "The Substitution of Hospital Outpatient Care for Inpatient Care," *Review of Economics and Statistics,* May 1972.

12. Evans, Robert G. "Efficiency Incentives in Hospital Reimbursement." Ph.D. dissertation, Harvard University, 1970.

13. Feldstein, Martin S. *Economic Analysis for Health Services Efficiency.* Chicago: Markham, 1968.

14. ———. "Hospital Cost Inflation: A Study of Non-Profit Price Dynamics." *American Economic Review* 61 (December 1971); 853–72.

15. ———. *The Rising Cost of Hospital Care.* Washington: Information Resources Press, 1971.

16. Feldstein, Paul J. "Research on the Demand for Health Services." *Milbank Memorial Fund Quarterly,* July 1966 (part 2).

17. Holtmann, A.G., "Prices, Time and Technology in the Medical Care Market."

18. Klarman, Herbert. "Approaches to Moderating the Increases in Medical Care Costs, *Medical Care,* May-June 1969.

19. ———. "Comment." *Empirical Studies in Health Economics,* ed. Herbert E. Klarman, pp. 315–320. Baltimore: Johns Hopkins University Press, 1970.

20. ———. "Reimbursing the Hospitals: The Differences the Third Party Makes," *Journal of Risk and Insurance,* December 1969.

21. ———. "Policy Alternatives for Controlling Health Services Expenditures." Paper presented at A.E.A. meeting, December 1970.

22. Lave, Lester, and Lave, Judith. "Hospital Cost Functions," *American Economic Review* 60 (June 1970): 379–395

23. New York State Department of Labor. *Employment Statistics.* Albany, 1968.

24. Newhouse, Joseph. "Toward a Theory of Non-Profit Institutions: An Economic Model of a Hospital." *American Economic Review* 60 (March 1970):64–74.

25. Pauly, Mark V., and Drake, David F., "The Effect of Third-Party Methods of Reimbursement on Hospital Performance." In *Empirical Studies in Health Economics*.

26. Rafferty, John A., "Patterns of Hospital Use: An Analysis of Short-Run Variations." *Journal of Political Economy*, January-February 1971.

27. Rosenthal, Gerald. *The Demand for General Hospital Facilities.* Chicago: American Hospital Association, 1964.

28. Russell, Louise B., "A Cost Model of Medicare." Ph.D. dissertation, Harvard University, 1971.

29. Sales Management Inc., *Survey of Buying Power*, annual.

30. Salkever, David. "Studies in the Economics of Hospital Costs." Ph.D., dissertation, Harvard University, 1970.

31. U.S. Bureau of the Census. *City and County Data Book: 1967.*

32. ———. *Census of Population: Characteristics of the Population*, vol. I, part 34. Washington, D.C., 1963.

33. U.S. Bureau of Labor Statistics, *Handbook of Labor Statistics: 1968*. Washington, D.C., 1968.

Hospital Wage Inflation: Supply-Push or Demand-Pull?

Rapidly rising wages were one of the prominent features of the hospital industry's cost-inflation spiral during the 1960s. While the average cost per day of inpatient care increased at an annual average rate of 9.7 percent over the decade, the average annual earnings of hospital employees rose by 6.2 percent yearly.[1] The corresponding rate of increase in the average hourly earnings of all private nonagricultural employees was only 4.4 percent. Rates of increase in weekly or hourly earnings for virtually all hospital occupations exceeded the general pace of wage inflation in the economy.[2] The gap between hospital and nonhospital wages for similar jobs had narrowed very considerably by the end of the decade.[3]

In spite of its importance in the cost-inflation process, the rapid rise of wages has not been systematically analyzed in the literature on hospital-sector inflation. There has been some discussion of the demand-pull theory—that rising wages were caused primarily by the growing demand for hospital services[4]—but alternative theories have not been considered in any detail. More significant is the lack of empirical studies designed to test these explanations of wage inflation.[5] The present study attempts to partially fill these voids.

To be specific, I shall test two alternative explanations of wage inflation: the demand-pull theory and the supply-push theory—that wage inflation was caused by economywide labor-market trends that radically altered the labor-supply conditions confronting the hospitals. Empirical analysis will be restricted to the wages of unskilled female employees. Besides being numerically important,[6] this group should be more responsive than technically trained personnel in hospital-specific jobs to changing labor-market conditions. Analysis of wage increases for this group should therefore provide a clear test of the effects of general labor-market trends. Furthermore, as Edelson has noted, the "philanthropic wage-setting" variant of the demand-pull theory[7] would presumably be most important for these unskilled workers because they are the lowest paid of all hospital employees.[8]

Although this study focuses on wage inflation per se, it has implications for understanding cost inflation. In several recent and important studies Martin Feldstein has argued that the rapid rise in hospital costs was primarily the result of an increased demand for hospital care.[9] He contends that increased demand led to higher costs partly because hospitals responded by raising wages "philanthropically" to "higher-than-necessary" levels. In this chapter Feldstein's view of cost inflation will be tested in two ways. First, I examine the empirical validity of Feldstein's conjectures about the relationship of rising demand to rising wages. Second, by testing the theory that general labor-market trends were a cause of wage inflation, it will indicate whether Feldstein's demand-oriented view of cost inflation should be broadened to include inflationary pressures from the supply side. In addition, this test of his theory has implications for wage inflation in other industries as well. If general labor-market trends led to relative wage gains in the hospitals, they may have had similar effects in other industries.

In the second, third, and fourth sections I develop and test specific hypotheses relating to the demand-pull and supply-push theories. First, however, I shall briefly describe the temporal and geographic pattern of wage increases.

The Temporal and Geographic Pattern of Wage Increases

Table 3–1 clearly shows the rapid pace of wage inflation for unskilled female hospital workers relative to the rise in nonhospital wages. In 1960 the average hourly wages of hospital maids for the fifteen SMSAs shown were only three-fourths of the wages of female janitors, porters, and cleaners in all industries. By 1969 the wages of the two groups were almost equal on average. It is also clear that the pace of catching up was uneven. Only a small relative wage increase occurred from 1960 to 1963; the increases for both 1963–1966 and 1966–1969 were somewhat larger.[10]

Substantial variation exists among areas in the extent of relative wage increases. In southern areas, especially Baltimore and Memphis, large increases occurred; by contrast, gains in the West Coast SMSAs and in Minneapolis were quite small. As shown in table 3–2, a similar pattern of regional variation existed for metropolitan areas in general over the 1963–1969 period. Relative wage gains were smallest in the West, moderate in the Northeast, and largest in the South and North Central regions. Overall it appears that the increases were greatest in areas where hospital wages were relatively low and least where hospital wages were relatively high.[11]

The Supply-Push Theory of Hospital Wage Inflation

According to the supply-push theory, relative wage gains for unskilled hospital workers were the result of cyclical and secular changes in the

Table 3–1
**Wages of Hospital Maids Relative to Female Janitors, Porters,
and Cleaners in All Industries: Selected SMSAs**

SMSA[a]	July 1960	July 1963	July 1966	March 1969
Atlanta	0.60	0.58	0.79	0.89
Baltimore	0.70	0.70	0.83	1.03
Boston	0.83	0.85	0.92	1.11
Buffalo	0.78	0.81	0.92	0.99
Chicago	0.69	0.71	0.74	0.90
Cincinnati	0.72	0.76	0.88	0.97
Cleveland	0.73	0.79	0.81	0.96
Dallas	0.73	0.83	0.90	0.95
Memphis	0.56	0.67	0.86	0.97
Los Angeles	0.79	0.78	0.75	0.84
Minneapolis	0.93	0.96	0.98	0.99
New York	0.74	0.86	0.91	1.03
Philadelphia	0.67	0.68	0.83	0.93
San Francisco	0.77	0.78	0.81	0.88
Portland (Ore.)	0.85	0.84	0.86	0.86
Average of 15 SMSAs	0.74	0.77	0.85	0.95

Source: The all-industry wage data are from the Bureau of Labor Statistics' Area Wage Surveys and were interpolated to coincide with the timing of the BLS hospital wage surveys. Hospital wage data are from the 1960, 1963, and 1969 BLS hospital industry wage surveys. The 1960 survey is reported in U.S. Bureau of Labor Statistics, *Earnings and Supplementary Benefits in Hospitals, Mid-1960*, Bulletin No. 1294 (Washington, D.C.: U.S. Government Printing Office, 1961).

Note: The figures shown are the ratio of the mean straight-time hourly wages for hospital maids to the mean straight-time hourly wages for female janitors, porters, and cleaners in all industries. Hospital maids' wages for 1963, 1966, and 1969 apply to short-term nongovernmental hospitals. Data for 1960 apply to all nonfederal short-term hospitals.

[a] Area definitions do not always correspond to SMSA definitions. See table 1A–1 for a listing of these area definitions.

labor market during the 1960s. These changes caused a narrowing of interindustry wage differentials for unskilled workers, or in other words, an increase in the unskilled wage level in low-wage industries relative to the corresponding level for all industries. Relative gains for hospital workers resulted because the hospital industry supply curve of unskilled labor is closely and positively related to the wage level of low-wage industries. But what cyclical and secular labor-market changes produced this result?

One such change may have been pronounced cyclical tightening of the labor market which produced a decline in unemployment rates from 6.7 percent in 1961 to 3.5 percent in 1969. Wachter's recent work suggests that this led to a narrowing of interindustry wage differentials, particularly for unskilled workers.[12] According to his argument, low-wage industries

Table 3–2
Wages of Hospital Maids Relative to Female Janitors, Porters, and Cleaners in All Industries: Metropolitan Area Averages

Area	1963	1966	1969
United States	0.80	0.83	0.92
Northeast	0.85	0.87	0.94
South	0.74	0.82	0.91
North Central	0.79	0.82	0.92
West	0.85	0.88	0.89

Source: The all-industry wage data are from the following U.S. Bureau of Labor Statistics publications: *Wages and Related Benefits: Metropolitan Areas, United States and Regional Summaries 1962–63*, Bulletin No. 1345-83, Part II (Washington, D.C.: U.S. Government Printing Office, 1964); *Wages and Related Benefits: Metropolitan Areas, United States and Regional Summaries 1965–66*, Bulletin No. 1465-86, Part II (Washington, D.C.: U.S. Government Printing Office, 1966); *Area Wage Surveys: Metropolitan Areas, United States and Regional Summaries 1968–69*, Bulletin No. 1625-91 (Washington, D.C.: U.S. Government Printing Office, 1970).

Note: The average hospital wage figures used in computing the ratios in this table are from the 1963, 1966, and 1969 Bureau of Labor Statistics hospital industry wage surveys and apply to nonfederal short-term hospitals in all metropolitan areas.

bid up wages in the competitive labor market as labor demand increases and unemployment falls. But this wage increase does not lead to inadequate supplies of labor for high-wage industries (operating in noncompetitive labor markets) because their workers are paid a premium above competitive-market wages. Furthermore, since these high-wage industries prefer to pursue acyclical wage-setting policies, they do not raise wages in response to a cyclical increase in competitive-market wages. The result is that wages in low-wage industries catch up during periods of low unemployment and fall back, relative to wages in high-wage industries, when employment returns to normal levels.

Two types of noncyclical changes in labor-market conditions—increases in the level of welfare payments[13] and declines in the extent of racial discrimination[14]—may also have narrowed wage differentials. There are several mechanisms by which this could occur. First, since rising welfare payment levels increase the attractiveness of leisure, and since a decline in discrimination undoubtedly diminished the "crowding" of nonwhites into the unskilled market,[15] a decline in the total supply of unskilled labor probably resulted. In terms of Wachter's framework, this would imply a rise in competitive wages for unskilled workers. Furthermore, because this rise is secular rather than cyclical in nature, employers in noncompetitive labor markets would respond by lowering their secular wage premiums,[16] and a secular narrowing of interindustry differentials in unskilled wages would result.

Second, rising welfare payments and declining discrimination would lead to secular narrowing of wage differentials if interindustry segmentation is present in the market for unskilled labor. In the jargon of dual-labor-market theory, there may be primary and secondary markets for unskilled labor, with the latter including hospital workers. Workers in this secondary market would be more strongly affected by rising levels of available public assistance because their attachment to their jobs (and to the labor force) is casual.[17] Similarly, the supply-reducing effects of the decline in racial discrimination would also be more important in the secondary market if discrimination had previously made it difficult for nonwhites to obtain primary market jobs.[18] These arguments imply a long-run increase in unskilled wages in the secondary market relative to the primary market, because the reduction in unskilled labor supply was greater in the former.

In summary, I hypothesize that declining discrimination and rising welfare payments brought about relative wage increases for unskilled female hospital employees. They produced this result by an increase in competitive-market wages relative to noncompetitive wages (according to the Wachter-Ross formulation) or an increase in secondary-market wages relative to primary-market wages (according to the dual-labor-market formulation). I also hypothesize that declining unemployment rates during the 1960s contributed to this relative wage inflation. Empirical tests of these hypotheses are reported in the fourth section of this chapter.

These supply-push hypotheses apply not just to hospitals but to all low-wage industries. If they are correct, relative wage gains for unskilled female workers should be observed in other industries besides hospitals. Evidence on this point is considered in the fifth section.

The Demand-Pull Theory of Wage Inflation

Undoubtedly, the demand for hospital care rose very rapidly during the 1960s. The main source of this increase was the growth in hospital insurance coverage, which reduced the fraction of expenses paid for directly by the consumers of hospital services. From 1960 to 1968 the fraction of total hospital expenses paid for directly by consumers fell from 0.286 to 0.158.[19] Of course, other factors such as rising real per capita income and technological progress in medicine also contributed to this growth in demand.

According to the demand-pull theory, rapidly rising wages resulted from this increase in product demand. Several explanations could be offered in support of this theory.

First, increased product demand induces hospitals to expand employment.[20] If the supply curve of unskilled female labor to the hospital industry is upward sloping (in either the short run or the long run) over the relevant range, this expansion in employment can be achieved only by raising hospital wages relative to nonhospital wages.

Second, rising demand greatly improved the overall financial status of hospitals. According to Feldstein's philanthropic wage-setting hypotheses, hospital management passed on some of the benefits of this improvement to unskilled workers in the form of higher-than-necessary wages. They may have done this for purely charitable reasons or perhaps because they felt a social obligation to pay decent or just wages. But whatever the reason, they willingly paid wages above the levels required to attract the desired supply of labor.

Feldstein's own statement of his hypothesis suggests that this behavior is indeed consistent with the social role of hospitals.

> The simplest economic logic requires that a profit-seeking firm should try to hire whatever group of workers it wants at lowest possible cost. . . . The same principle is not at all compelling to the management of a nonprofit institution. A hospital, as a philanthropic or public organization, may concern itself with the welfare of its staff as well as of its patients. The tradition of low pay for hospital staff developed when hospital budgets were very tight and the institutions were largely dependent on voluntary philanthropic support. More recently, the rapid rise in the demand for hospital care has given hospital administrators much greater freedom in determining salary levels . . . hospitals could, and I believe have, used their increased discretionary financial power . . . by raising the wages of hospital personnel above the levels necessary to obtain the staff they wanted.[21]

A third explanation is that rising demand and the consequent improvement in the financial status of hospitals led to wage increases because it intensified employee pressures for these increases. Edelson has argued that this hypothesis is more appealing than the philanthropic hypothesis because it is consistent with more conventional and realistic assumptions about the motivations of hospital managers.

> An alternative to the charity hypothesis is that improved finances have increased wages because of pressure from employees. Such pressures can be manifested in various ways: union demands; threats to unionize; or excessive quit rates. This more conventional view of wage determination is supported by the motives generally imputed to non-profit institutions; whether hospitals are viewed as maximizing a utility function that

has as its arguments the quantity and quality of ''output'', or whether they are viewed as instruments for maximizing physicians' incomes, hospitals will never voluntarily pay workers more than the going wage.[22]

One might question the generality of this employee-pressure hypothesis, however. Where a formal or informal organization of employees exists, these pressures—communicated in the form of union demands or threats to unionize—are backed by the market power of this organization. Where it does not exist, employee pressures would not be effective unless management responded to them in an effort to reduce the risk of future organizing efforts. Even if this is the case, it still seems reasonable to expect that the response to employee pressures will be greater in places where employees are organized.

These considerations suggest that rising product demand raised relative wages indirectly, through increases in employment, and/or directly as suggested by the philanthropic and employee-pressure hypotheses. The next section first attempts to measure this effect of rising demand and then tests the hypothesis that its magnitude is related to the presence of employee organization.

Empirical Tests of the Supply-Push and Demand-Pull Theories

Specific hypotheses relating to the demand-pull and supply-push theories will be tested with cross-sectional time-series data on a group of large SMSAs by estimating the parameters of the following type of relative-wage-determination equation:

$$RW_{it} = F(X_{1it}, \ldots, X_{kit}; Z_1, \ldots, Z_n; e_{it})$$

where the X's are explanatory variables relating to the hypotheses, the Z's are SMSA-specific dummy variables, e_{it} is an error term, and RW_{it} is the wage of hospital maids relative to female janitors, porters, and cleaners in all industries in the ith SMSA in year t.[23]

The X's that relate to supply-push hypotheses set forth in the second section are[24]

U_{it} (−) = average annual unemployment rate in the ith SMSA in year t

W_{it} (+) = real average monthly AFDC money payment per recipient

R_{it} (+) = ratio of nonwhite to white median annual earnings of female workers[24]

U is included to test the hypothesis that cyclical changes in labor-market conditions accounted for part of the increase in RW. W relates to the hypothesis that rising welfare payments caused relative wage gains while R is included to measure the impact of declines in labor-market discrimination. R is a useful summary measure of discrimination because it is affected by a variety of differences between white and nonwhite workers that may be manifestations of discrimination. These include differences in occupational distributions, differences in unemployment rates, and differences in weeks and hours worked.[25]

To test the demand-pull theory, we shall include several explanatory variables whose changes over time can serve as proxies for changes in the level of demand for hospital services. That is, we can define a level-of-demand parameter D as being derived from the demand function for hospital services, denoted by $Q_{DH} = Dp^n$, and we can interpret the demand-pull hypotheses in terms of a relationship between increases in D and increases in RW. Furthermore, note that D is a function of a variety of demand-affecting variables such as insurance coverage and income. Since we cannot observe D directly, we include these variables as proxies for D in the relative-wage-determination equation:

M_{it} (+) = real expenditures per inhabitant on medical assistance payments

H_{it} (+) = percentage of the population with hospital insurance coverage

I_{it} (+) = per capita real income

That these variables are all proxies for D indicates that the magnitude of their effects on RW should be related to the magnitude of their effects on D. Since numerous empirical studies have indicated that the demand for hospital services is far more sensitive to variations in insurance coverage than variations in income, we would expect H to have a greater positive effect than I on RW.[26] Similarly, H should have a greater effect than M, which is intended to measure the insurance coverage of a small segment of the population, welfare recipients and medically needy persons. Finally, only M, H, and I are included on the assumption that other variables affecting D could be presumed constant over the period 1963–1969 within each SMSA. The effects of these other variables are therefore included in the estimates of the dummy-variable coefficients.

We shall also perform an additional test relating specifically to the rising derived-demand explanation of demand-pull. To be specific, we shall test the assumption of an upward-sloping labor supply curve to the hospital industry in an area, on which this explanation is based, by including the following as an explanatory variable.

E_{it} (+) = ratio of unskilled female employment in hospitals to total unskilled female employment in the SMSA[27]

In addition to omitted demand variables, a fully-specified model of relative-wage determination would probably include many other variables, not considered in this study, relating to supply and demand conditions and to market structure in the market for unskilled labor. The inclusion of SMSA dummy variables will permit unbiased estimation of coefficients for the included explanatory variables provided that the combined effect of these omitted variables on RW (for any given values of the included variables) has not changed over time within any SMSA.[28]

Log-linear and linear relationships between RW and the explanatory variables (with the Z's also included) were estimated by OLS using three cross sections of observations on fifteen large SMSAs.[29] The 1963 cross section included twelve of the areas shown in table 3–1.[30] The 1966 and 1969 cross sections included these same twelve areas plus Detroit, St. Louis, and Washington.[31]

Table 3–3 presents results obtained with a log-linear specification when both supply-push and demand-pull variables were included in the estimated equations.[32] In general, results for individual variables are rather unstable, indicating the presence of multicollinearity in the data. Evidence for several of the supply-push hypotheses appears stronger than that for the demand-pull hypothesis, but the sample does not contain sufficient information to reach any definitive conclusions.

When all explanatory variables are included (equation 3.1), the estimates conflict with the hypotheses in several ways. The coefficients of U and H have the wrong signs while none of the remaining variables except R and I even approaches significance. Furthermore, the highly significant coefficient for I is not consistent with the restriction, implied by the demand-pull hypothesis, that it should not exceed the coefficient of H.[33] When this restriction is incorporated into the estimation process (equations 3.7–3.11), the estimates provide stronger confirmation of the supply-push hypotheses relating to rising welfare payments and declining discrimination. Also the coefficient of H becomes positive and nearly significant when restricted to equality with the coefficient of I (equations 3.7–3.9). But when it is restricted to being twice as large as the coefficient of I, its significance declines. Since the latter restriction seems more consistent with the demand-pull hypothesis[34] the evidence for that hypothesis appears weak. Similar conclusions about the hypotheses emerge when the coefficient of I is restricted to zero (equations 3.2 and 3.3).

Because the results cast doubt on the demand-pull hypothesis, I have also estimated relative-wage-determination equations that include only supply-push variables (table 3–4).[35] These equations support my previous findings that R and W are valid explanations of relative wage inflation and

Table 3–3
Log-Linear Regression Results: Supply-Push and Demand-Pull Variables
(*t-statistics in parentheses*)

Equation	R	W	U	H	M	I	E	R^2
3.1	0.323 (1.22)	0.095 (0.83)	0.139* (1.43)	-0.312 (0.57)	0.037 (0.82)	0.741** (1.97)	0.041 (0.32)	0.893
3.2	0.552** (2.17)	0.119 (0.98)	0.011 (0.15)	-0.026 (0.05)	0.028 (0.60)	—	0.032 (0.25)	0.872
3.3	0.525** (2.48)	0.124 (1.12)	—	-0.032 (0.06)	0.027 (0.61)	—	—	0.872
3.4	—	0.152 (1.17)	-0.069 (0.93)	0.514 (0.95)	0.084** (1.92)	—	-0.004 (0.03)	0.844
3.5	—	0.154 (1.25)	-0.068 (0.96)	0.511 (0.97)	0.083** (2.00)	—	—	0.844
3.6	—	0.235** (1.91)	-0.113* (1.58)	1.220** (2.97)	—	—	—	0.817
3.7	0.332 (1.22)	0.136 (1.19)	0.072 (0.82)	0.364* (1.33)	0.022 (0.49)	0.364[a]	-0.004 (0.04)	0.882
3.8	0.311 (1.21)	0.123 (1.18)	—	0.251 (1.11)	0.025 (0.58)	0.251[a]	—	0.878
3.9	0.397** (1.92)	0.132 (1.30)	—	0.257 (1.16)	—	0.257[a]	—	0.877
3.10	0.404* (1.48)	0.138 (1.18)	0.040 (0.49)	0.362 (0.91)	0.021 (0.46)	0.181[b]	-0.021 (0.17)	0.877
3.11	0.439** (2.07)	0.142* (1.39)	—	0.313 (0.91)	—	0.157[b]	—	0.874

Note: All regressions include a constant term and fourteen SMSA dummies. The value of R^2 in a regression including only the constant and these dummies was 0.443.

[a]Restricted to be equal to the coefficient of H.

[b]Restricted to be 0.5 times the coefficient of H.

*90 percent significant, one-tailed test.

**95 percent significant, one-tailed test.

Table 3-4
Log-Linear Regression Results: Supply-Push Variables Only

Equation	R	W	U	E	R^2
4.1	0.639**	0.139*	0.015	—	0.870
	(4.71)	(1.32)	(0.21)		
4.2	0.617**	0.136*	—	—	0.870
	(7.48)	(1.33)			
4.3	0.629**	0.131	—	−0.024	0.870
	(6.07)	(1.21)		(0.20)	
4.4	—	0.218*	−0.254**	—	0.749
		(1.55)	(4.14)		

Note: All regressions include a constant term and fourteen SMSA dummies. The value of R^2 in a regression including only the constant and these dummies was 0.443.

*90 percent significant, one-tailed test.

**95 percent significant, one-tailed test.

that, contrary to expectations, tightening labor markets were not important in this inflation process. The coefficient of U has the correct sign and is significant only when R is excluded from the analysis (equations 3.6 and 4.4).[36] However, in view of the collinearity problems, a conclusive rejection of the tightening-labor-markets hypothesis is not possible.

The coefficient of E is insignificant in all regressions,[37] implying that the long-run hospital industry supply curve of unskilled female labor is horizontal.[38] Increased derived demand does not seem to have been an important factor in relative wage inflation.[39]

The final set of results concerns the demand-pull theory and the relationship of employee organization to rising product demand. To test the hypothesis that a greater degree of organization increases the effect of demand on wages by increasing the effectiveness of employee pressures, I divided the SMSAs into three groups according to the extent of organization and then reestimated several log-linear equations allowing for separate demand-pull effects for each group.[40] The results shown in table 3-5 indicate that the demand-pull effect does not vary monotonically with the extent of organization as hypothesized but is greatest where organization is present but not widespread (group 3). Since it is also true that union-organizing activity was somewhat greater over the 1963–1969 period in group 3 SMSAs than in the other groups, one is tempted to conclude that this result indicates the use of discretionary financial power to raise wages in response to the threat of unionization.[41]

As to the quantitative significance of the hypotheses for the wage-inflation process, two questions arise. First, how much of the overall increase in relative wages is explained by the estimated equations? That

Table 3–5
Log-Linear Regression Results: Employee Organization Effects

Equation	R	W	H1	H2	H3	M1	M2	M3	R^2
5.1[a]	0.556** (2.30)	0.065 (0.68)	-0.275 (0.51)	-0.465 (0.79)	0.554* (1.73)	-0.040 (0.43)	0.039 (0.56)	-0.010 (0.22)	0.930
5.2[a]	0.377** (4.37)	0.106* (1.32)	—	—	0.738*** (4.16)	—	—	—	0.924
5.3[b]	0.720** (3.17)	0.028 (0.26)	-1.181 (0.78)	-2.146 (0.80)	0.514 (1.05)	-0.012 (0.08)	0.083 (0.59)	-0.002 (0.04)	0.922
5.4[b]	0.414** (4.27)	0.019 (1.21)	—	—	0.708* (1.55)	—	—	0.046 (1.29)	0.910

Note: All regressions include a constant term and fourteen SMSA dummies. The value of R^2 in a regression including only the constant and these dummies was 0.443.

Coefficients of H_1 and M_1 are coefficients for the ith group of SMSAs.

[a]The coefficient of I is restricted to equal 0.5 times the coefficient of H for each group of SMSAs.

[b]I is excluded; the coefficients of the H_i are unrestricted.

*90 percent significant, one-tailed test.

**95 percent significant, one-tailed test.

is, do these equations track the movement of relative wages closely? Or
do they overpredict in 1963 and underpredict in 1969, thereby leaving
much of the 1963–1969 increase unaccounted for? And second, which
particular variables were most important in explaining this increase?

To answer the first question, I computed the mean predicted values
for RW in 1963 for equations 3.5, 3.9, 4.2, and 4.9 and obtained values that
were in all cases almost identical to the actual mean R of 0.778. I then
performed the same calculation for 1969 and obtained figures that never
deviated by more than 0.007 from the actual mean RW of 0.958. These
results indicate that a very large fraction of the increase in RW is in fact
explained by these equations.

Unfortunately, the second question cannot be answered because of
collinearity problems. The importance of any one variable will vary
widely as other variables are introduced or deleted from the regression
equation. However, the coefficients of equation 3.11 (which includes both
demand-pull and supply-push variables) imply that the increase in RW due
to declining discrimination was twice as large as the increase in RW due to
rising demand and five times as large as the increase due to rising W.[42]

In summary, the results tend to confirm that secular changes in the
market for unskilled labor, brought about by declining discrimination and
rising welfare payments, were important causes of relative wage gains for
hospital workers. On the other hand, there was little support for the
hypotheses that the cyclical tightening of the labor market also contributed to these gains. Evidence for the demand-pull theory was also rather
weak, especially with regard to the hypothesis that rising derived demand
increased wages. There were some indications, however, that the effect of
demand on wages is more positive in areas where employees are not
extensively unionized but the threat of unionization is present.

Further Evidence on the Supply-Push Theory

While the results of the empirical analysis generally indicate that the
supply-push theory explains an important part of observed relative wage
inflation, some additional evidence must be examined before we accept
this conclusion. According to the supply-push theory, relative wage gains
in the hospital industry were part of a general process of narrowing
interindustry wage differentials for unskilled workers throughout the
economy. If the theory is correct, this process should be evident in other
industries as well as in hospitals. Although the supply of relevant published data is rather meager, it does indeed contain such evidence.[43]

Table 3–6 indicates the extent of relative wage gains in the laundry
and cleaning industry. For the country as a whole these gains were fairly

Table 3–6
Wages of Female Inside-Plant Laundry Workers Relative to
Female Janitors, Porters, and Cleaners in All Industries:
Metropolitan Area Averages

Region	June 1963	April 1968
United States	0.77	0.83
Northeast	0.82	0.87
South	0.79	0.86
North Central	0.76	0.82
West	0.85	0.83

Sources: U.S. Bureau of Labor Statistics, *Industry Wage Survey: Laundry and Cleaning Services, June 1963,* Bulletin No. 1901 (Washington, D.C.: U.S. Government Printing Office, 1964); *Industry Wage Survey: Laundry and Cleaning Services, April 1967 and April 1968,* Bulletin No. 1645 (Washington, D.C.: U.S. Government Printing Office, 1969); *Wages and Related Benefits: Metropolitan Areas, United States and Regional Summaries 1962–63,* Bulletin No. 1345–83, Part II (Washington, D.C.: U.S. Government Printing Office, 1964); *Wages and Related Benefits: Metropolitan Areas, United States and Regional Summaries 1967–68,* Bulletin No. 1575-87, Part II (Washington, D.C.: U.S. Government Printing Office, 1969).

Note: Figures are ratios of mean straight-time hourly earnings.

substantial though not as large as in the hospital industry (see table 3–2). Furthermore, the geographic pattern of wage gains was similar to that for hospitals. In fact, the ranking of regions by the magnitude of these gains is identical for the two industries, although the regional variation is somewhat greater for hospitals.

Table 3–7 presents similar data for contract cleaning services and again shows clear evidence of relative wage gains. In this case, however, the gains were fairly small in all regions except for the South.

Finally, CPI data on the wages of domestic workers provides additional supporting evidence. Over the 1961–1970 period the CPI figure for domestic services increased by 65.8 percent. Over the same period the average wage of female janitors, porters, and cleaners in all industries rose by only 44.9 percent. The 46.4 percent rise in the CPI figure for domestics over the 1963–1969 period is comparable to the 53.6 percent increase for hospital maids' wages over this same period.[44] This similarity between wage increases for domestic workers and hospital workers is of particular interest because relative wage gains for domestic workers probably cannot be explained by factors such as unionization and changes in minimum wage laws, which may have had some effects in other industries.[45]

In short, although the evidence from other industries is sparse it does tend to confirm the supply-push theory. It indicates that the wages of

Table 3–7
Wages of Female Cleaners in Contract Cleaning Relative
Female Janitors, Porters, and Cleaners in All Industries:
Metropolitan Area Averages

Region	1961	1968
Northeast	0.92	0.96
South	0.87	1.02
North Central	0.94	0.96
West	1.00	1.02

Sources: U.S. Bureau of Labor Statistics Area Wage Surveys for each of these SMSAs and the following BLS publications: *Industry Wage Survey: Contract Cleaning Services, Summer 1961*, Bulletin No. 1327 (Washington, D.C.: U.S. Government Printing Office, 1962) and *Industry Wage Survey: Contract Cleaning Services, July 1968*, Bulletin No. 1644 (Washington, D.C.: U.S. Government Printing Office, 1969).

Note: Figures are ratios of mean straight-time hourly earnings. They are averages of ratios for the following SMSAs: *Northeast:* Boston, Newark and Jersey City, New York, Philadelphia, Pittsburgh; *South:* Atlanta, Dallas, Miami, Washington; *North Central:* Chicago, Cleveland, Detroit, Milwaukee, Minneapolis, and St. Paul, St. Louis; *West:* Los Angeles and Long Beach, San Francisco and Oakland, Seattle.

unskilled female workers in most low-wage industries (including the hospital industry) were catching up throughout the economy, as a result of the labor-market forces identified.

Concluding Comments

There are several implications of these results. They suggest that the widely accepted demand-oriented view of recent hospital cost inflation should be broadened to include at least a modicum of inflationary pressures from the supply side. This is not to dispute the obvious fact that the hospital industry's response to increased demand resulted in higher costs. But it points out that contrary to the implications of the demand-oriented view, at least some cost inflation was beyond the control of the hospitals.

This observation is of some importance in the context of the current health policy emphasis, at both state and federal levels, on regulatory control of hospital costs. Determined regulatory resistance to inflationary pressures that are beyond the control of the hospitals may cause serious difficulties. More specifically, if labor-market trends continue to cause upward shifts in the supply curve of unskilled labor to hospitals, and if hospital wages cannot respond to this shift because of regulatory controls, shortfalls in labor quantity or quality will result. Although this problem might be alleviated in the long run by adjustments in the hospitals' production processes, short-run deterioration of services would be likely.

The confirmation of several of the supply-push hypotheses points to the existence of similar inflationary pressures in other sectors. This is confirmed by the bits of evidence presented in the fifth section, but a more thorough analysis of labor markets in other labor-intensive industries experiencing rapid inflation is called for.

Finally, the limitations of this analysis and its results also bear repeating. We have examined only wage inflation for unskilled female employees, and the generalizing of conclusions to the case of skilled hospital employees is certainly not warranted. Indeed, even for unskilled female employees the limited amount of information in the sample data implies that the conclusions are decidedly tentative. Further research is clearly needed to obtain a definitive and comprehensive understanding of the recent hospital wage inflation.

Notes

1. See U.S. Social Security Administration, Office of Research and Statistics, *Medical Care Costs and Prices: Background Book*, DHEW Publication (SSA) 72-11908, January 1972, pp. 26–27.

2. In other words, the rapid rise of hospital wages was not merely a reflection of a changing occupational mix in the hospital work force. See Martin Feldstein, *The Rising Cost of Hospital Care* (Washington, D.C.: Information Resources Press, 1971), chap. 5, and Noel Edelson, "The Influence of Skill Mix, Monopsony Power, and Philanthropy on Hospital Wage Rates," Discussion Paper No. 211, Department of Economics, University of Pennsylvania, 1971.

3. A useful summary of statistics on hospital wage inflation is provided in Feldstein, *Rising Cost of Hospital Care*, chap. 5. See also tables 3–1 and 3–2 in this chapter.

4. Feldstein, *Rising Cost of Hospital Care*, chap. 5, and Edelson, "Influence of Skill Mix."

5. The only available empirical studies are Karen Davis "Theories of Hospital Inflation: Some Empirical Evidence," *Journal of Human Resources* 8 (1973): 181–201, "Hospital Costs and the Medicare Program," *Social Security Bulletin* 38 (1973): 18–86, and Edelson, "The Influence of Skill Mix." These studies suffer from potentially important defects in specification. For example, Edelson does not include any variables directly relating to the demand for hospital services; nor does he include any variables relating to labor-market conditions that may effect the relationship between hospital and nonhospital wage rates for similar occupations. This latter omission also occurs in Davis's work.

6. 1969 Bureau of Labor Statistics data indicate that this group makes up 31 percent of all full-time nonsupervisory hospital employees. This figure is derived from U.S. Bureau of Labor Statistics, *Industry Wage Survey: Hospitals, March 1969*, Bulletin No. 1688 (Washington, D.C.: U.S. Government Printing Office, 1971), pp. 3, 15.

7. The notion of philanthropic wage-setting was formulated in Feldstein, *Rising Cost of Hospital Care,* pp. 67–69, and is explained in the third section.

8. See Edelson "Influence of Skill Mix," p. 17. On the other hand, the industry supply elasticity is presumably high for this group of workers, so the inflationary impact of rising derived demand will be difficult to detect. This is less likely to be true for skilled employees, such as nurses and technicians.

9. See Feldstein, *Rising Cost of Hospital Care,* chap. 3; "Hospital Cost Inflation: A Study in Nonprofit Price Dynamics," *American Economic Review* 61 (1971): 853–872; and "The Quality of Hospital Services: An Analysis of Geographic Variation and Intertemporal Change," Discussion Paper No. 279, Harvard Institute of Economic Research, 1973.

10. However, table 3–2 indicates that for metropolitian areas in general the increases for 1963–1966 were considerably less than those occurring in 1966–1969.

11. This pattern is consistent with the view that hospital wage inflation of the 1960s was merely a catching up to equilibrium wage levels defined by equality with nonhospital wages. Estimates of lagged adjustment models that lend some support to this view are presented in Edelson, "Influence of Skill Mix." But this interpretation is not very appealing for several reasons. First, hospital wages have been relatively low for decades, and it is doubtful that adjustment lags are that slow. Alternatively, there is no reason to believe that the recent decline in long-standing wage shortfalls in hospitals is due to slackening of a steady stream of inflationary shocks to nonhospital wages. Furthermore, given the possibility of equilibrium interindustry wage differences due to nonpecuniary differences, there is no compelling reason for believing that equilibrium hospital wages are equal to nonhospital wages even in an unsegmented, perfectly competitive labor market.

12. See M.L. Wachter "Cyclical Variation in the Interindustry Wage Structure," *American Economic Review* 60:75–84, and "Wage Determination in a Local Labor Market: A Case Study of the Boston Labor Market," *Journal of Human Resources* 7 (1972): 87–103.

13. In this chapter the level of welfare payments is measured by the average monthly payment per recipient to AFDC recipients (excluding medical vendor payments and recipients receiving only medical care). During the 1959–1969 period for the entire country this average payment increased by 66.0 percent, from $27.20 to $45.15. (See appendix 3A of this

chapter for the source of these figures.) Over the same period the CPI rose by only 25.8 percent.

14. For recent discussions of the decline in racial discrimination in the labor market, see R.B. Freeman, "Decline of Labor Market Discrimination and Economic Analysis," *American Economic Review* 63 (1973): 280–286, and Orley Ashenfelter, "Changes in Labor Market Discrimination over Time," *Journal of Human Resources* 5 (1970): 403–430.

15. The concept of racial discrimination as a process of crowding minority group members into less desirable occupations is developed in Barbara Bergman, "The Effect on White Incomes of Discrimination in Employment," *Journal of Political Economy* 79 (1971): 294–313. Freeman ("Decline of Labor Market Discrimination") suggests that much of this crowding may have occurred through extramarket (educational) discrimination rather than through discriminatory hiring practices in the labor market. Whatever the explanation, however, it is clear that nonwhites held a disproportionate share of low-skill jobs and that their relative occupational standing (especially for women) improved dramatically in the 1960s.

16. The reason for this can be inferred from the work of Ross and Wachter, which extends Wachter's original formulation. (See S.A. Ross and M.L. Wachter, "Wage Determination, Inflation, and the Industrial Wage Structure," *American Economic Review* 63 (1973): 675–692.) The secular wage premium generates a secular labor queue (or excess supply) in the noncompetitive sector, the function of this queue being to reduce the risk of productive capacity falling short of product demand. But secular increases in competitive unskilled wages make it more expensive to maintain a labor queue of a given size as insurance against excess demand. The result is that noncompetitive employers purchase less insurance; that is, they reduce the size of their desired queue for unskilled workers and lower the wage premium accordingly. See Ross and Wachter, "Wage Determination," pp. 678–681, for a more complete discussion of the noncompetitive firm's wage-setting decision.

17. This distinction between primary and secondary labor markets in terms of workers' attachments to specific jobs and the labor force in general has been discussed in Peter B. Doeringer and Michael J. Piore, *Internal Labor Markets and Manpower Analysis* (Lexington, Mass.: Lexington Books, D.C. Heath, 1971), chap. 8. It implies higher turnover rates in the secondary market. The extremely high turnover rates in hospitals suggests that it is indeed appropriate to include unskilled hospital workers in the secondary market.

18. In other jobs, this would be so if discrimination "crowded" nonwhites into unskilled jobs in certain industries rather than into unskilled jobs in general.

19. See Feldstein, *Rising Cost of Hospital Care*, table 2.5.

20. Increased labor inputs might be desired to expand output, to increase product quality, and/or to increase slack. There is at least some evidence that the expansion in unskilled employment was relatively rapid. For example, the numbers of full time maids, female kitchen helpers, and female nurse's aides all increased by over 10 percent from 1966 to 1969, while from 1965 to 1969 the total number of employed female service workers and female nonfarm laborers in the economy increased by only 4 percent. (See U.S. Bureau of Labor Statistics, *Industry Wage Survey: Hospitals, June 1966*, Bulletin No. 1553 (Washington, D.C.: U.S. Government Printing Office, 1967) and *Industry Wage Survey: Hospitals, March 1969*.)

21. Feldstein, *Rising Cost of Hospital Care*, p. 68. Reprinted with permission.

22. Edelson, "Influence of Skill Mix," p. 21. Reprinted with permission.

23. RW_{it} corresponds to the ratios shown in table 3–1. For its precise definition see table 3–1, note.

24. The signs in the parenthesis following the variables' names are the expected directions of their effects on RW_{it}.

25. A more detailed description of sources and definitions for all variables used in this study is given in appendix 3A.

26. Consider insurance a percentage reduction in the out-of-pocket cost of hospital care, and let c denote the percentage of the price that insured persons pay out of pocket; then the average net price in any particular area is equal to $P_G(H \cdot c + 1 - H)$, where P_G is gross price and H is the fraction of the population with coverage. If plausible values are assumed for c and H, the elasticity of average net price with respect to H might be as large as 2.0. Combining this fact with Feldstein's result ("Hospital Cost Inflation") that the price elasticity of demand for hospital services is more than twice as large as the income elasticity implies that the elasticity of RW with respect to H should be perhaps three or four times the corresponding income elasticity.

27. The coefficient of E measures the slope of the long-run supply curve. I also tested the assumption that the short-run curve has a nonzero slope by including the change in E as an explanatory variable.

28. The inclusion of the SMSA dummies also implies that coefficients of the explanatory variables measure the effects of time-series variation rather than cross-sectional variation in these variables. The use of pooled data is therefore based on the assumption that these time-series effects are the same across SMSAs.

29. It is likely that the OLS estimate of the coefficient for E is asymptomatically biased downward because of simultaneity. However,

since this coefficient provides only a supplemental test of one specific form of the demand-pull theory, I did not attempt to obtain consistent estimates by specifying a larger structural system.

30. Cincinnati, Memphis, and Portland were omitted because data on H were unavailable.

31. Regression results based on an expanded sample for equations not containing H as an explanatory variable are presented in table 3B–2.

32. Results based on a linear specification are shown in table 3B–1.

33. See the third section. Because of this inconsistency, the significantly positive coefficient for K should be regarded as a spurious result rather than a confirmation of the demand-pull hypothesis.

34. See note 26 for an explanation of this point.

35. The analogous linear equations are B1.6–B1.9 in table 3B–1. Linear and log-linear results with an expanded sample are shown in table 3B–2.

36. The only results at variance with this conclusion are in equations B2.1 and B2.2. However, the change in the coefficient of U when R is excluded does imply that R is itself affected by cyclical conditions. If cyclical changes in R were cointrolled for, more significantly negative coefficients for U would probably be obtained.

37. The only possible exception is equation B2.2 in table 3–2, where it is almost 90 percent significant.

38. When E was replaced by the change in E in linear regressions, and when the logarithm of E was replaced by its change in log-linear regressions, coefficient estimates were either negative or positive and clearly insignificant. This implies that the short-run supply curve is also horizontal within the observed range of variation.

39. Other explanations are possible, however. The within-SMSA year-to-year instability in the Bureau of Labor Statistics estimates of unskilled hospital employment point to the possibility of substantial measurement error. Also OLS estimates of the coefficient of E (or the logarithm of E) are biased downward because of simultaneity.

40. The groupings were (1) little or no organization: Dallas, St. Louis, Washington; (2) widespread organization: Minneapolis, New York, San Francisco; and (3) an intermediate extent of organization: the nine remaining SMSAs. These groupings were based on data on the extent of collective bargaining contract coverage for nonprofessional hospital workers (excluding office and clerical workers) from U.S. Bureau of Labor Statistics, *Industry Wage Survey: Hospitals, June 1966*, pp. 4–5 and *Industry Wage Survey: Hospitals, March 1969*, pp. 4–5. Notice that each SMSA was placed in the same group for 1963, 1966, and 1969. No attempt was made to measure changes in the extent of organization within an SMSA over this period because the BLS data are not sufficiently reliable or comprehensive to be used in that way.

41. Caution is required, however, because this result is somewhat fragile. When an alternative but also plausible grouping was used, in which Atlanta and Baltimore were placed in group 1, the coefficient of $H1$ also became positive and in some cases moderately significant. This result would be consistent with the interpretation if the threat of unionization was present even in group 1 SMSAs. But the sensitivity of the results to the grouping employed indicates the hazards of generalizing from information on only fifteen SMSAs.

42. The increase due to a particular variable was estimated by using coefficient estimates to calculate the change in the values of RW that would have occurred for 1969 if the variable in question had not changed in value from 1963 to 1969. The differences between these values of RW and the observed 1969 values measure the increase in RW due to that variable.

43. Ideally, one would like to examine occupation-specific wage data from a number of other competitive or secondary-market industries to see whether they experienced relative wage inflation similar to that in the hospital industry. This type of data has been published by the Bureau of Labor Statistics for a few of these industries.

44. The source of this figure is U.S. Bureau of Labor Statistics, *Industry Wage Survey: Hospitals, Mid-1963*, Bulletin No. 1409 (Washington, D.C.: U.S. Government Printing Office, 1964), table 2, and *Industry Wage Survey: Hospitals, March 1969, table 4*.

45. Increased unionization and minimum-wage laws have frequently been cited as explanations of wage inflation but are not considered in detail in this chapter for several reasons. The extent of unionization among hospital employees did not grow rapidly during the 1960s. For example, Bureau of Labor Statistics data show no change in the national percentage of nonprofessional hospital employees under collective bargaining from 1966 to 1969. The available evidence for the 1960–1966 period also does not indicate a general pattern of rapid increases in unionization. As Feldstein suggests (*Rising Cost of Hospital Care*, pp. 65–66), growth of unionization may be in part a response to growth in product demand rather than an exogenous cause of wage inflation. Rapid wage inflation occurred even in areas, such as Dallas, where unionization was virtually absent from any section of the hospital industry.

The effect of minimum-wage-law coverage of hospitals (in February 1967) does not appear to have been large in view of the facts that relative wage gains were already occurring and that for each SMSA in this study 1966 and 1969 average wages were well above the legal minimum. Of course, the impact of minimum wage levels in rural areas was probably greater.

Appendix 3A
Data Sources and
Definitions

This appendix briefly describes the principal sources and definitions of the data used in this study.

Hospital and Nonhospital Wages. Hospital wage data were taken from Bureau of Labor Statistics (BLS) hospital industry wage surveys. Nonhospital wage data were gathered from the BLS Area Wage Surveys and interpolated to coincide with the timing of the hospital wage surveys. Area definitions, which apply to both hospital and nonhospital wage data, are shown in table 3A–1.

Unemployment Rates. Data on total unemployment rates are from various editions of *The Manpower Report of the President* and relate to "major labor market-areas" as defined by BLS. Estimated rates corresponding to the 1969 area definitions in table 3A–1 were used for Memphis (1960), Cincinnati (1960 and 1963) and Cleveland (1960 and 1963) because published BLS data did not correspond to these area definitions. New York City data are for the five boroughs and were obtained from the New York State Department of Labor.

Welfare Payments. Data on average monthly money payments per AFDC recipient in the state in which the SMSA is located were taken from the public assistance statistics releases published monthly by the U.S. Department of Health, Education, and Welfare. Adjustments in published data were made to correct for the inclusion of recipients who received only medical assistance in the denominators of figures for money payments per recipient.

Consumer Prices. Per capita income and welfare payments data were deflated by indexes of living costs derived from BLS indexes of comparative living costs and from consumer price indexes published in the BLS *Handbook of Labor Statistics*. Estimated living cost figures for Buffalo (1960 and 1963), Dallas (1960 and 1963), Miami (1966 and 1969), Memphis (all years), and Portland (all years) were obtained from regression equations.

Ratios of Nonwhite to White Earnings. For 1969, the ratio of nonwhite earnings to white earnings was calculated from data for each SMSA on

Table 3A–1
Area Definitions for Bureau of Labor Statistics Wage Surveys

SMSA	Years	Counties Included
Atlanta	1960–1969	Clayton, Cobb, Dekalb, Fulton and Gwinnett Counties, Ga.
Baltimore	1960–1966	Baltimore City, Anne Arundel, Baltimore, Carroll, and Howard Counties, Md.
	1969	Add: Harford County, Md.
Boston	1960–1969	Suffolk County and parts of Middlesex, Essex, Norfolk, and Plymouth Counties, Mass.
Buffalo	1960–1969	Erie and Niagara Counties, N.Y.
Chicago	1960	Cook County, Ill.
	1963–1969	Add: Du Page, Kane, Lake, McHenry, and Will Counties, Ill.
Cincinnati	1960–1963	Hamilton County, Ohio, and Campbell and Kenton Counties, Ky.
	1966–1969	Add: Clermont and Warren Counties, Ohio, Boone County, Ky., and Dearborn County, Ind.
Cleveland	1960–1963	Cuyahoga and Lake Counties, Ohio
	1966–1969	Add: Geauga and Medina Counties, Ohio
Dallas	1960–1966	Collin, Dallas, Denton, and Ellis Counties, Tex.
	1969	Add: Kaufman and Rockwell Counties, Tex.
Denver	1966–1969	Adams, Arapahoe, Boulder, Denver, and Jefferson Counties, Col.
Detroit	1966–1969	Macomb, Oakland, and Wayne Counties, Mich.
Los Angeles	1960–1969	Los Angeles and Orange Counties, Cal.
Memphis	1960–1963	Shelby County, Tenn.
	1966–1969	Add: Crittenden County, Ark.
Miami	1966–1969	Dade County, Fla.
Minneapolis	1960–1969	Anoka, Dakota, Hennepin, Ramsey, and Washington Counties, Minn.
New York	1960–1969	Bronx, Kings, New York, Queens and Richmond Counties, N.Y.
Philadelphia	1960	Philadelphia and Delaware Counties, Pa. and Camden County, N.J.
	1963–1969	Add: Bucks, Chester, and Montgomery Counties, Pa. and Burlington and Glouchester Counties, N.J.
Portland	1960–1969	Clackamas, Multnomash, and Washington Counties, Ore. and Clark County, Wash.
San Francisco	1960–1963	Alameda, Contra Costa, Marin, San Francisco, San Mateo, and Solano Counties, Cal.
	1966–1969	Delete: Solano County
Saint Louis	1966–1969	St. Louis City, Franklin, Jefferson, St. Charles, and St. Louis Counties, Mo. and Madison and St. Clair Counties, Ill.
Washington, D.C.	1966	District of Columbia, Montgomery and Prince Georges Counties, Md.; Alexandria, Fairfax, and Falls Church Cities and Arlington and Fairfax Counties, Va.
	1969	Add: Loudoun and Prince William Counties, Va.

white and black female median earnings from the 1970 census series *Detailed Social and Economic Characteristics*, table 195. Data from 1960, 1963, and 1966 were obtained by first computing ratios of nonwhite to white earnings (from the 1960 census series *Detailed Social and Economic Characteristics*, table 124) and then interpolating the 1959–1969 change in this ratio over the intervening years in proportion to the changes in the national ratio reported in *Current Population Reports: Series P-60*, no. 69 (table A-7) and no. 75 (table 62). New York City data for 1959 and 1969 are for the five boroughs.

Income. Per capita income figures for each SMSA (and for the five boroughs of New York City) are those prepared by Sales Management, and published in their *Annual Survey of Buying Power*.

Hospital Insurance Coverage. Data on the percentage of the population covered by hospital insurance in each SMSA for 1963 are those for fiscal 1963 published by the National Center for Health Statistics (NCHS). For 1969 unpublished NCHS estimates for calendar 1968 were employed. Data for 1966 were interpolated from these NCHS figures in proportion to the 1963, 1966, and 1968 percentages for the states in which the SMSAs are located. These state percentages were derived from state population figures published in the *Statistical Abstract*, from figures on numbers of persons covered by hospital insurance published annually in Health Insurance Association of America, *Sourcebook of Health Insurance Data*, and (for 1968) from Social Security Administration data on Medicare enrollment.

Real Medical Assistance Payments per Capita. Data for 1966 and 1969 on state per capita spending for public assistance medical vendor payments were obtained from the calendar 1966 and fiscal 1969 issues of *Trend Report: Graphic Presentation of Public Assistance Data* published by the Social and Rehabilitation Service, U.S. Department of Health, Education, and Welfare. Corresponding data for 1963 were obtained from the annual statistical supplement to the journal *Welfare in Review*, published by the same agency. Data for 1969 were then deflated by the spring 1969 comparative indexes of costs for medical care calculated by the Bureau of Labor Statistics. Data for 1963 and 1966 were also deflated by these indexes after being inflated to 1969 price levels as indicated by the CPI medical care component.

Employment Ratios. Nonfederal hospital employment figures representing the sum of full-time maids, female kitchen helpers, nurse's aides, and psychiatric aides were obtained from the BLS hospital industry wage surveys. Minor adjustments in these figures were then made, for some SMSAs and some years, to obtain employment estimates specifically for short-term hospitals and to correct for changing area definitions on the BLS surveys. Total unskilled female employment for each area, which we estimated as the sum of service workers (household and nonhousehold) and nonfarm laborers, was obtained from 1960 census data for 1960. Estimates for later years were linear interpolations of the 1960 and 1970 census figures.

Appendix 3B
Additional Empirical Results

Table 3B–1 presents regression results, for a linear specification, of equations analogous to some of those shown in tables 3–3 and 3–4. Table 3B–2 presents regression results for equations that include supply-push variables but no demand-pull variables except E. These are based on data for four cross sections (1960, 1963, 1966, and 1969) and twenty SMSAs. The fifteen SMSAs shown in table 3–1 are included in all four cross sections, while 1966 and 1969 data also include Denver, Detroit, Miami, St. Louis, and Washington.

Table 3B–1
Linear Regression Results

Equation	R	$W \times 10^{-2}$	$U \times 10^{-2}$	$H \times 10^{-2}$	$M \times 10^{-3}$	$I \times 10^{-3}$	E	R^2
B1.1	0.458**	0.361	0.574	−0.049	−0.636	0.126*	0.485	0.893
	(1.93)	(1.24)	(0.33)	(0.09)	(0.51)	(1.39)	(0.34)	
B1.2	0.617**	0.351	−0.668	0.214	−0.864	—	0.213	0.883
	(2.91)	(1.18)	(0.43)	(0.40)	(0.68)		(0.15)	
B1.3	0.665**	0.355	—	0.215	−0.801	—	—	0.881
	(3.72)	(1.27)		(0.42)	(0.67)			
B1.4	—	0.566*	−2.754**	1.250**	−0.489	—	0.494	0.836
		(1.70)	(1.75)	(2.68)	(0.33)		(0.29)	
B1.5	—	0.495**	−2.783**	1.213**	—	—	—	0.834
		(1.96)	(1.88)	(3.02)				
B1.6	0.642**	0.222	−0.645	—	—	—	—	0.880
	(4.65)	(0.99)	(0.45)					
B1.7	0.685**	0.237	—	—	—	—	—	0.879
	(7.05)	(1.08)						
B1.8	0.680**	0.239	—	—	—	—	0.139	0.879
	(6.26)	(1.07)					(0.10)	
B1.9	—	0.537**	−5.349**	—	—	—	—	0.771
		(1.85)	(3.82)					
B1.10	—	—	—	0.65	1.087	0.230**	0.470	0.857
				(0.31)	(1.06)	(3.62)	(0.31)	
B1.11	—	—	—	1.514**	1.886*	—	0.541	0.775
				(3.22)	(1.54)		(0.29)	

Note: All regressions include a constant and fourteen SMSA dummies. The value of R^2 in a regression including only the constant and these dummies was 0.451

*90 percent significant, one-tailed test.

**95 percent significant, one-tailed test.

Table 3B–2
Expanded Sample Regression Results

Equation	Functional Form	R	W	U	E	R^2
B2.1	Linear	0.547** (4.55)	$0.422** \times 10^{-2}$ (1.91)	$-1.938* \times 10^{-2}$ (1.46)	—	0.833
B2.2	Linear	0.506** (4.04)	$0.445** \times 10^{-2}$ (2.02)	$-1.870* \times 10^{-2}$ (1.41)	1.236 (1.12)	0.834
B2.3	Log-linear	0.638** (5.66)	0.216** (2.24)	-0.012 (0.18)	—	0.857
B2.4	Log-linear	0.655** (10.58)	0.218** (2.30)	—	—	0.856
B2.5	Log-linear	0.637** (8.19)	0.226** (2.31)	—	0.033 (0.38)	0.857

Note: All regressions include a constant and nineteen SMSA dummies. Linear and log-linear regressions including only the constant and these dummies yielded R^2 values of 0.363 and 0.362 respectively.

*90 percent significant, one-tailed test.

**95 percent significant, one-tailed test.

4

Measuring the Impact of Prospective Rate Setting: An Overview of Recent Econometric Research

The effectiveness of regulation has been a dominant theme in recent empirical work on hospital costs. Interest in this subject was stimulated by increased federal and state reliance on hospital investment and revenue controls. Several Blue Cross plans have also implemented new investment and rate-review mechanisms. Federal research funding agencies have recently given a high priority to evaluative research on these regulatory programs, and their investment (while modest in dollar terms) has yielded a number of new studies. This chapter seeks to provide a detailed but concise review of methods and findings from several of these studies. Most of the discussion concerns studies of prospective rate-setting programs operated by individual states or by Blue Cross plans. According to Bauer, the defining characteristic of these programs is that "the amounts to be paid for specified units of service are established by some external authority prior to the period in which the services are to be given."[1] Typically these amounts have been defined as per diem rates for inpatient-days, although the use of per case rates is now gaining favor. The prospective per diem rates have usually been established either by applying an inflation factor to previous years' per diem rates (or costs) or by determining a hospital's projected total expenditures and volume of patient-days, with the ratio of projected expenditures to projected days being the prospective per diem rate.[2]

Recent econometric research on the impact of the federal Economic Stabilization Program (ESP) will also be reviewed. This program, which was in effect from August 1971 to April 1974, differed slightly from Bauer's definition of prospective reimbursement. It established upper limits on prices or revenues for each hospital rather than setting specific rates or revenue levels. Nevertheless, since new federal revenue limitation programs are now being actively considered,[3] the experience under the ESP program is of considerable interest.

This chapter consists of four sections. To place the review of specific studies in a larger context, the first section considers the rationales for using various impact measures in assessing the success or failure of rate-setting programs. I suggest that the choice of impact measures should be based primarily on performance criteria for the entire health care system rather than on the stated objectives of the regulatory programs under study. A variety of impact measures are discussed, including several that have often been overlooked in studies to date. The next two sections describe the methods, results, and limitations of the studies of prospective rate-setting and ESP programs. The emphasis here is on techniques and quantitative findings rather than on interpretation. The concluding section discusses the interpretation of findings and directions for future research.

Impact Measures of Hospital Rate-Control Programs

Perhaps the most critical element in any study of a rate-control program's effectiveness is the choice of impact measures (dependent variables). This choice can substantially influence the degree of success or failure attributed to a program. More important, it specifies the criteria by which success or failure will be defined. Obviously these criteria should correspond directly to the objectives set for the program. However, the precise nature of these objectives is not so obvious.

Objectives of Rate-Control Programs

Several views of the objectives of rate-control programs can be distinguished. The narrowest is that these programs should increase hospital efficiency in producing each unit of service. If efficiency gains are achieved, any given volume, mix, and quality level of hospital services can be produced with fewer inputs of real resources and hence less opportunity cost. But to operationalize the objective of increased efficiency, units of service must be defined. These could be defined broadly, such as a day of inpatient care, treatment of an inpatient case, or an outpatient visit. Alternatively specific types of services could be identified—laboratory tests, diagnostic x-ray procedures, meals served, and so on.[4] The definition of units of service determines whether reductions in various types of hospital utilization achieved by a rate-control program are viewed as pure efficiency gains. With a broad definition of units of service, reductions in ancillary utilization (say, laboratory tests or radiology procedures) that led to lower costs per inpatient-day or per case would represent efficiency gains. Moreover, if the unit of inpatient service is defined as the case rather than the day, reductions in average length of stay would also imply increased efficiency. But these reductions in utilization would not constitute an increase in efficiency if units of service are defined in very specific terms (tests, procedures, meals). With such specific definitions, hospital efficiency could be increased only by improving productive efficiency of the departments within the hospital.

A more inclusive objective for a rate-control program is to reduce the total costs of hospital care (or the total resources used in providing hospital care) for the entire population of a defined geographic area. This objective is based on the premise that excessive hospital costs are due both to inefficiency in producing each unit of service and to excessive use of hospital services.[5] Reductions in inpatient admissions per capita, inpatient-days per capita, or outpatient visits per capita achieved by a rate-control program contribute to this objective even if they do not increase the efficiency of individual hospitals.

An even broader objective for a rate-control program is to reduce total health care costs, including costs incurred by both hospital and nonhospital providers of care. This objective might be preferable to the preceding ones because of the recognition that a rate-control program could reduce hospital costs by shifting hospital services to nonhospital settings, thereby increasing the total cost of nonhospital care. If this occurs, the real resource savings achieved by the program will be less than the savings observed in the hospital sector. Such shifts of health care resource to less tightly regulated settings seem quite likely in light of past experience with regulation elsewhere.[6] That these shifts are technically feasible and potentially significant has been illustrated by the recent growth of ambulatory surgical facilities and of computed tomography installations in physician's offices.[7]

Which of these objectives is most important for policymakers in judging the success or failure of a rate-control program? To answer this question, first consider the narrower objective of increasing hospital efficiency and assume that increases in efficiency are indicated by reductions in cost per inpatient-day or per case. Of course, reductions in cost per day resulting from the implementation of a rate-control program could be achieved simply by extending length of stay, thus increasing the total cost of hospital care.[8] Similarly reductions in cost per case could be achieved by admitting additional patients merely for diagnostic work or simple surgical procedures previously performed in an ambulatory setting, again resulting in higher total hospital costs.[9] Conversely, reductions in length of stay and shifting of some short-stay admissions to outpatient settings could lead to higher costs per day and per case respectively, though in each instance total hospital costs would presumably decline.

The lesson to be drawn from these examples is that improvements in hospital efficiency as indicated by reductions in cost per day or cost per case are a very uncertain guide to the success or failure of a rate-control program. What matters for policy purposes is the economic performance of the entire hospital sector or the entire health care system in the geographic area under study. Economic performance is gauged by total resource costs and by effectiveness in promoting the health of the population.[10] Clearly the two broader objectives of controlling total hospital costs or total health care costs are more consistent with this view. It follows that a rate-control program's success is best measured by its impact on total hospital costs and total health care costs rather than its effect on cost per day or per case.[11]

But one might contend that these broader goals of total cost containment should not be applied in evaluative studies because rate-control programs are in fact intended to achieve only the narrower goal of increasing hospital efficiency. Explicit statements of this narrower goal are typically found in the relevant legislation and administrative guidelines.[12] This contention is bolstered by the recent spread of other regulatory programs—Professional Standards Review Organizations (PSROs) and certificate-of-need investment controls—directed primarily at controlling excessive hospital utilization. Where these other programs are operating to control the quantity of hospital services provided, a reasonable division of regulators' labor would seem to require that a rate-control program focus primarily on the unit cost of services.[13]

Two points should be considered in response to this argument. First, if one accepts the basic premise that control of total costs is the ultimate policy concern, then program evaluations that do not assess total cost impacts can have only limited significance in the policymaking process. Whether one accepts this premise is, of course, a subjective matter. However, it is clearly consistent with the recent trend in policy proposals toward explicit ceilings on total expenditure or revenue such as those contained in the Carter administration's cost-control bill and in the "maxicap" programs being implemented in Rhode Island and upstate New York.[14] Second, the presence of other regulatory programs seeking to limit the quantity of services does not eliminate the need to assess total cost impacts but rather affects their interpretation. The operation of these programs in the same geographical area as a rate-control program precludes the statistical estimation of total cost impacts for the rate-control program per se when the control areas have no regulatory programs in operation. Instead, one can only estimate the combined impact of both types of regulation in the experimental areas.[15] If the control areas do have some form of quantity regulation, it may be possible to estimate the total cost impact of adding a rate-control program, but this poses special methodological problems.[16]

Rationales for Various Types of Impact Measures

Thus far I have argued that evaluation studies ought to focus on the broader objectives of controlling total health care costs or total hospital costs, even though they are not the explicitly stated objectives of a rate-control program, and that the program's measured impact on total costs is the principal indicator of its success. However, to judge the program's effect on the economic performance of the health care system, we must also consider its impact on that system's effectiveness in maintaining and promoting population health levels. Unfortunately, this impact is often extremely difficult to determine, and various proxy measures for it are often employed. Now we merely note that in determining whether a rate-control program was successful, attention must be paid to health impacts as well as cost impact. If total costs are reduced with no decline in the effectiveness of care, a clear gain in system efficiency has been achieved. If a program reduces both costs and effectiveness of care, a judgment as to its success depends on societal values as interpreted by decision makers in the policy making process; the issue cannot be settled within the confines of evaluative research.

Of course, the overall economic performance of the health care system is not the only concern for policymakers. The achievement of equity goals has also been a major theme in health policy formulation.[17] In particular, a variety of governmental programs such as the National Health Service Corps and the Neighborhood Health Centers program have been enacted to increase accessibility to services by disadvantaged or "underserved" population groups. Cost-control programs may also influence accessibility, but it seems likely a priori that this influence will be adverse to the attainment of equity goals. If costs are controlled by cutting back on "unnecessary" and duplicative services, there is a good chance that these cutbacks will affect primarily the disadvantaged and underserved who are least able to defend their interests in the regulatory process. This suggests that it is important to measure the effect of a rate-control program on access to care for these population groups. The indicators of access used in this measurement could include quantities of various types of services used or process measures of access, such as waiting times for elective hospital admissions or travel and waiting time for obtaining ambulatory services.[18]

Measures of impacts on total health care costs, population health levels, and equity of access are useful for judging whether a rate-control program has improved the performance of the health care system and therefore whether the program is a success or a failure. But often limitations of data and technique require the use of proxies for these measures. For example, impacts on total health care costs are usually difficult to measure because data on the costs of services of private physicians and other nonhospital providers are not readily available. Data on the costs of hospital services are plentiful but represent only 45 percent of national health care costs.[19] Insurance benefit payments for nonhospital services could be used as a proxy for the costs of these services, but such payments reflect only services consumed by insured persons (rather than by the entire population of the area) and exclude the costs of deductibles, coinsurance, charges in excess of fee schedules, and noninsured services.[20] Utilization measures (numbers of doctor visits or days of nursing home care) could also be used as proxies, but reliable state-level or small-area data on nonhospital utilization are sparse. Other proxy measures may be useful because of the limited time frame of an evaluative study. For instance, impacts on hospital investment or capital stock are indicative of future effects on hospital operating costs that cannot be observed within the time span of a study. Impacts on net revenues or liquid assets of hospitals have also been interpreted this way. In particular, Berry has suggested that hospitals may react initially to the budgetary restrictions of a cost-control program by running losses and drawing down reserves but that a deterioration in their financial position eventually requires cuts in expenditures.[21] As this observation implies, the proxies for future cost impacts suggested here are especially useful for evaluations of rate-control programs that have been operating for only a short time.[22]

Proxy measures are even more necessary in assessing health impacts. Direct measurement of program impact on population health levels (as indicated by various mortality and morbidity data) is extremely difficult because so many other factors affect health levels and because often we cannot control for enough of these other factors to accurately gauge the presumably small effect of rate controls.[23] Moreover, there may be a considerable time lag before any program effects are revealed in mortality and morbidity data. The standard practice has consequently been to fall back on "process" indicators of medical care quality. In this approach medical records (or abstracts of records) for selected groups of hospital patients are examined to determine the fraction of cases in which the care provided conformed with professionally determined standards of good practice.[24] The assumption underlying this exercise is that if a rate-control program caused a decline in the quality of care (in frequency of conformance to standards of good practice), this would result in poorer outcomes of care and lower population health levels. However, empirical support for this assumption is often not available. Furthermore, many of the studies that I shall review do not even attempt to examine medical care process impacts, relying instead on cruder measures or ignoring the quality issue (and hence the health impact issue) altogether.[25]

Still other impact measures may be of interest, not as indicators of whether a rate-control program worked, but because they aid in understanding how it functioned. Included here are effects on hospital efficiency as indicated by impacts on cost per day or per case or by estimated shifts in hospital production functions. Some studies examine departmental-level data to determine cost impacts in particular departments. This allows a test of the proposition that cost savings will be greater in departments controlled by the administration (nursing, laundry, housekeeping) than in departments controlled primarily by the medical staff (such as laboratory and ancillary service departments).[26] Impacts on hospital utilization—length of stay, number of admissions, diagnostic mix of admissions—are of interest since they indicate whether hospital admitting and discharge policies have been affected by the rate-control program. Impacts on investment or capital stock (numbers of beds, availability of specialized facilities) also give a more detailed picture of how a rate-control program affects hospitals, though these impacts serve the additional purpose of being proxies for longer-run effects on costs not observable within the study period. Simple descriptive measures of program operations can provide further insight. Examples of such measures include the extent to which regulators reduce allowable rates below the levels requested by hospitals and the frequency and amount of incentive payments or penalty assessments in programs with special incentive or penalty features.

These impact measures are of interest from a broad public policy perspective; other measures of program impact may be of interest to particular organizations or agencies. Third-party payors, for example, will be particularly interested in rate-control impacts on the quantity and cost of services delivered to the populations that they cover. Planning agencies may be especially concerned with impacts on utilization of various types of services and investment in new facilities and services. Manpower policymakers are likely to be interested in impacts on hospital staffing levels and patterns. In short, there are many potentially important effects of rate-control programs that have been overlooked in this discussion but which researchers (and the sponsors of research) may wish to examine.

Summary and a Concluding Comment

Before turning to the empirical research, a brief summary of the discussion thus far will be helpful. The success or failure of a rate-control program should be judged by its impact on the performance of the health care system. The three dimensions of performance of utmost concern for public policy are total costs, maintenance or improvement of population health levels, and equity of access. Thus program impacts on total costs, health levels, and equity of access should be regarded as the most appropriate success indicators. However, proxies for these impacts may be needed because of limitations of data and of the time span of the research. Other impact measures, such as those pertaining to hospital efficiency and utilization, are of interest for understanding how a rate control program works. A variety of measures may be of interest to particular organizations or agencies even though these measures may receive little weight in health policy decisions relating to rate-control programs.

Finally, though I have argued that the measures used to judge a program's success need not correspond to the program's explicit objectives, it does not follow that these objectives are irrelevant for the researcher. Statements of objectives may indicate the particular variables or concerns that attract the most attention in the regulatory process. Similarly, they may be viewed as guidelines to which regulators' decisions are expected to adhere. If so, these objectives provide information about the way a program functions and suggest hypotheses about its strengths and weaknesses that can be tested in the course of the research.

Research on Prospective Rate Setting

This section reviews five studies that examined the rate-setting programs in Indiana, New Jersey, New York State (upstate and downstate), and Rhode Island. These studies were carried out under contracts with the Division of Health Insurance Studies, Office of Research and Statistics, Social Security Administration, and the Department of Health, Education, and Welfare.[27] Since the same set of technical specifications applied to all five contracts[28] and, as a result, to federal efforts to coordinate the work of these contractors, the methods employed in all five studies were quite similar. This review is confined to the impact measures used in the studies, the methods of estimating these impacts, and the statistical significance and magnitude of the estimated impacts. Other issues addressed in the studies—the costs of administering the rate-setting programs, administrative processes and problems, and the potential for implementing such programs in other states—are not considered here.

Descriptions of the Rate-Setting Programs

Rhode Island. Prospective rate setting by Blue Cross in Rhode Island began in fiscal year 1971 (October 1, 1970, to September 30, 1971).[29] Rates for one large hospital were determined in a budget review and negotiation process, while rates for all other hospitals were simply based on their submitted budget requests. From projected expenditure and volume figures, a routine inpatient per diem rate, a nursery per diem rate, delivery room charges, and a rate for outpatient visits were calculated. Charges for ancillary services were computed as a percentage markup of these routine service rates. Hospitals were at risk for added costs above these rates and could keep 50 percent of actual costs below these rates if actual volume figures for the various types of services fell within predetermined ranges of their volume projections. If actual volumes fell outside these ranges or if other unforseen special circumstances caused actual costs to exceed projections, rates could be renegotiated. In fact, during fiscal 1971 two hospitals experienced financial problems because of inaccurate utilization estimates, and six of the thirteen hospitals in the program requested renegotiations.

The fiscal 1971 prospective rates appear to have been rather generous, since they were based on total budget increases of 12.9 percent for the one negotiated budget and 16.5 percent on average for the other twelve hospitals. In fiscal 1972 an effort was made to increase the stringency of controls. All hospitals' Blue Cross rates were determined by budget review and negotiation. The state hospital association entered the process by organizing preliminary budget reviews for each hospital carried out by committees of administrators and trustees from other hospitals. Hospital representatives also served, along with Blue Cross representatives, on a mediation committee that resolved impasses in the 1972 budget negotiations between Blue Cross and four of the hospitals. The outcome of the 1972 process was the approval of budgets which were, on average, about 13 percent greater than the actual fiscal 1971 total expenditure levels.

Though the Rhode Island program was limited to setting rates for Blue Cross patients, more than 80 percent of the state's population is covered by Blue Cross. Moreover, the fraction of patients covered by the program increased during its second phase (which began in fiscal 1975) when the Medicaid and Medicare programs also became participants in the process.[30]

New Jersey. A program of prospective budget review began in New Jersey in 1969 under the auspices of the Commissioner of Banking and Insurance.[31] This initial review activity was limited to twenty high-cost hospitals that were expected to exceed the 1969 ceiling on per diem Blue Cross payments set by the commissioner. Per diem rates in excess of the ceiling, which these hospitals were seeking, could be approved only through the prospective review process. Presumably because the year-to-year increases in the ceiling rates did not keep pace with hospital-sector inflation, an additional forty-three hospitals entered the review system in 1970, and eighteen more hospitals entered in 1971. The Health Facilities Planning Act enacted by the state legislature in May 1971 gave the commissioner of health authority to set Medicaid rates and shared responsibility (with the commissioner of insurance) for approving hospital charges to Blue Cross. Thus by 1973, when all New Jersey hospitals had voluntarily entered the budget review system, the rates for Blue Cross, Medicaid, and the other state-supported patients—accounting for 43 percent of all patient-days—were set through the budget review process.

The program determined all-inclusive per diem rates for each hospital. If actual per diem costs were less than these rates, however, hospitals were reimbursed only for their costs. Thus the program set a ceiling on rates but did not provide rewards (in the form of net revenue) for holding costs below this ceiling. If a hospital's per diem cost exceeded its prospective rate, it absorbed the loss unless a retroactive rate adjustment was approved by the commissioner of health.

Although the New Jersey program has always been an official state government function, until recently it relied heavily on assistance from the participating hospitals. Staff from the New Jersey Hospital Association's Hospital Research and Educational Trust (HRET) played the major role in reviewing budget submissions for the advisory committee to the comissioners of health and insurance. Advisory committee reviews were carried out by subcommittees on which hospital administrators and trustees were in the majority. Partly as a result of criticisms that the program had been captured by the hospitals,[32] the HRET role was eliminated in 1974 and the staff of the Department of Health assumed the review and analysis functions.

New York. Since 1970 three different rate-setting systems have been in operation in New York: one for Medicaid patients throughout the state, one for Blue Cross patients in the downstate (southeastern) portion of the state, and one for Blue Cross patients in the remainder of the state (upstate).[33] The Medicaid program is administered by the State Department of Health, while the downstate and upstate Blue Cross programs are administered by Greater New York Blue Cross and by a combination of the seven upstate Blue Cross plans respectively. Under the authority of the Hospital Cost Control Act of 1969, the Department of Health is responsible for supervising and approving the rates set in the Blue Cross programs.

The New York programs use a formula (rather than budget review) approach for determining an inclusive per diem rate for each hospital. The formula consists of a base cost computation and the application of a trend factor to this base cost. The base cost is calculated from the hospital's estimated actual costs in the current year or its actual costs of the preceding year. Hospitals are also grouped to compute ceilings on cost levels for the previous year and on rates of increases between current and previous years. If any hospital exceeds either of these ceilings, its computed base cost is reduced accordingly. Reductions are also made for hospitals that do not achieve minimum occupancy rates. Once the base cost is computed, it is multiplied by the trend factor that accounts for expected increases in wages and nonlabor input prices during the coming year.

The formula-determined rates are set annually and apply for a twelve-month period, but hospitals can appeal for higher rates. In particular, hospitals must appeal for inclusion of costs of new services, since no costs for these services are added to the base cost figure. Appeals to allow for increases in input prices (particularly wage settlements) that were not accurately reflected in the trend factors have been frequent. The heavy number of appeals has posed administrative problems and has often delayed determination of a hospital's rate until long after the beginning of the year to which the rate applies.

The hospital's incentives under this cost-based formula approach are rather unclear. In the short run a hospital reaps the benefits of costs below the per diem rate in the form of net revenue. But these lower costs will reduce the rate set for the hospital in subsequent years. Of course, uncertainty introduced by administrative delays in determining rates may alter these incentive effects.

Indiana. The Indiana rate-setting program differs from the other four programs under discussion in several important respects.[34] First, it has a long history. It was established in 1960 as a response by the Indiana Hospital Association and Indiana Blue Cross to public concerns about rising hospital costs. Until 1960 Indiana Blue Cross had paid hospitals their billed charges without prior review and approval of charge levels.

Second, it is a private sector effort with minimal involvement of the state government. The Rate Review Commission appoints its own members and is accountable (either formally or informally)[35] only to Indiana Blue Cross. While a number of hospital administrators or trustees are commission members, they are in the minority. The majority of members are physicians, business executives, academics, accountants, and other private citizens. The staff support for the commission is provided by Indiana Blue Cross.

Third, the rates set by the Indiana program are applied to self-paying patients and patients covered by other insurance companies as well as to Blue Cross beneficiaries. Excluding only Medicare and Medicaid patients, the Indiana program thus controls rates for 75 percent of hospital cases in the state, which account for over 60 percent of total revenues.

Hospitals submit annual rate proposals to the commission containing their revenue and volume projections. Proposed rates for all specific services and a daily room charge are specified in this submission, although the commission's review focuses primarily on total cost and revenue figures, labor costs, wage rates, or particular problem areas; a detailed review of rates for each of the specific services is not undertaken. Once rates have been approved for a hospital (either as proposed or modified to meet the commissions' objections), these rates are in effect for the subsequent twelve months. Any net revenues or losses resulting from unexpected volume variations or other factors accrue entirely to the hospital. However, emergency requests for rate increases can be made during the year (though this rarely occurs), and depletion of working capital due to losses can be used to justify higher rates in the following year.

Estimates of Cost Impacts

Estimates of cost impacts in all five studies were derived from regression analyses of hospital costs. In all studies the unit of analysis was the individual hospital, and the study sample included both experimental hospitals subject to rate setting and control hospitals from neighboring states that were not under rate controls.[36] Except in the Indiana study, data for years both before and after the implementation of rate setting were included. Average cost per day or per case was used as the dependent variable.[37]

Two important features of the regression models employed in these studies are the methods of specifying rate-setting program effects and the selection of control variables. One simple approach to measuring program effects is to estimate the linear model

$$C = \alpha_0 + \beta Z + \gamma T + \alpha_1 R + \delta RT \qquad (4.1)$$

where C is the cost variable, R is a dummy variable equal to one if a hospital is subject to rate setting, T is either a time trend or a vector of time variables (such as, dummy variables for individual years), and Z is the vector of control variables. In this model the effect of rate setting ($\alpha_1 + \delta T$) is assumed to vary with time. Although a standard F-test can be used for the null hypothesis that rate-setting has no effect ($\alpha_1 = \delta = 0$), a test for the magnitude of the rate-setting effect is more complicated. It requires computation of the standard error of the estimated effect, that is, $[\text{var}(\hat{\alpha}_1) + T^2 \text{ var}(\hat{\delta}) + 2T \text{ cov}(\hat{\alpha}_1, \hat{\delta})]^{1/2}$.[38] One suggested simplification is to estimate the regression

$$C = \alpha_0 + \beta Z + \gamma T + \alpha_2 R + \delta R(T - \bar{T}) \qquad (4.2)$$

where $\bar{T}$ is the mean value of T.[39] If the model specified in equation 4.1 is correct, then the true value of α_2 is ($\alpha_1 + \delta \bar{T}$), which is the effect of rate setting evaluated at the mean of T. Thus $\hat{\alpha}_2$ is the estimate of this effect, and its standard error can be used to compute a confidence interval (conditional on the assumption that $\hat{\delta} = \delta$). Of course this procedure is unnecessary for the simpler models in which the rate-setting effect is constant over time ($\delta = 0$) or is proportional to $T(\alpha_1 = 0)$, but the realism of such models may be questioned.

The effect of rate setting can also be estimated in the log-linear (double-log) model

$$\log C = \alpha_0 + \beta \log Z + \gamma T + \alpha_1 R + \delta RT \qquad (4.3)$$

Here one might assume that the effect of rate setting is constant in percentage terms ($\delta = 0$). Though this is more plausible than a constant absolute effect (as in the linear model with $\delta = 0$), it still seems restrictive.

A more complicated procedure used in several of the studies involves allowing for structural differences between control hospitals and experimental hospitals and for changes in these differences over time. This is illustrated by the linear model

$$C = \alpha_1 C_1 + \alpha_2 C_2 + \alpha_3 E_1 + \alpha_4 E_2 + \gamma_1 C_1 T + \gamma_2 E_2 T$$
$$+ \gamma_3 E_1 T + \gamma_4 E_2 T + \beta Z \quad (4.4)$$

where C_1 and C_2 are dummy variables denoting control hospitals before and after the advent of rate setting, respectively, and E_1 and E_2 are analogous dummy variables for experimental hospitals. The effect of rate setting in this model is the difference between the shifts in the α and γ coefficients after the introduction of rate setting for the experimental hospitals and the corresponding shifts for the control-hospital coefficients. This difference is equal to

$$(\alpha_4 - \alpha_3) - (\alpha_2 - \alpha_1) + (\gamma_4 - \gamma_3)T - (\gamma_2 - \gamma_1)T$$

Equation 4.4 may be rewritten as

$$C = \alpha_0^* + \alpha_1^*(E_1 + E_2) + \alpha_2^*(C_2 + E_2) + \alpha_3^* E_2 + \gamma_0^* T$$
$$+ \gamma_1^*(E_1 + E_2)T + \gamma_2^*(C_2 + E_2)T + \gamma_3^* E_2(T - \bar{T}) + \beta Z \quad (4.5)$$

where α_3^* equals the effect of rate setting as just defined when evaluated at the mean value of T. Thus the estimated coefficient $\hat{\alpha}_3^*$ measures this effect.[40] Finally, note that the model can be extended by allowing for differences in the β's between experimental and control hospitals and for differential shifts in the β's over time.

The vector of control variables Z is included in the model to account for specific influences on cost levels that may have differed between the control and experimental groups in the periods before or after the advent of rate setting. The econometric literature on hospital costs suggests two approaches to specifying these variables. One approach is based on the view that the regression model is an estimate of a technological or quasi-technological cost function (roughly analogous to the standard textbook cost function). This function relates the level of average cost to the volume of output, the mix of output, factor prices, and (in short-run cost functions) the rate of capacity utilization or the capital stock. The usual measures of output volume are patient-days or admissions, while capacity utilization is measured by the occupancy rate or case-flow rate (admissions per bed). Capital stock is typically represented by the number of beds in the hospital and often by indicators of the presence of special facilities and services. The latter variables may also be viewed as indicators of output mix. Other commonly used output mix variables are measures of outpatient services, teaching activity, the diagnostic mix of inpatients, and their average length of stay. Factor prices have often been accounted for by including wage rate variables, locational proxies for factor-price differences (such an urban-rural dummy), and price indices (such as the CPI or WPI).

The second approach is to estimate a behavioral cost equation. This equation treats observed cost levels as the result of a decision process in which hospital objectives are maximized subject to product market, factor market, and technological constraints. Explanatory variables typically include demand-influencing factors (such as the income and insurance coverage of the population in the area where the hospital is located), supply influences (such as wage rates), and hospital characteristics (such as ownership type) that are intended to control for differences in objectives among hospitals. It is also customary to view this equation as a short-run construct and thus to include capital stock variables as well.[41]

The interpretations of rate-setting effects differ in these two models. A negative rate-setting coefficient in the quasi-technological model indicates that any given volume and mix of output is produced with less cost as a consequence of rate setting. Presumably this reflects an increase in hospital efficiency. A similar coefficient in a behavioral model could be the result of greater efficiency, but it could also indicate changes in the actual volume and mix of output induced by the rate-setting program. This distinction implies a limitation of the quasi-technological model. The output measures used as explanatory variables in this model are themselves likely to be influenced by the rate-setting program, and the implication for average cost levels of this influence is not captured in the model. A similar comment applies to the capital stock variables in both models, however, since a rate-setting program may also affect hospital investment. Thus to obtain a more complete picture of the effects of rate-setting on costs, the impacts of rate setting on output and investment should also be examined. The studies reviewed here carried out such analyses.[42]

The control variables actually used in the five rate-setting studies are described in table 4–1. In three of these studies (New Jersey, downstate New York, and Rhode Island) the choice of variables corresponds closely to the quasi-technological approach. The other two studies (Indiana and upstate New York) combine selected variables from both approaches, so it is not clear which conceptual framework is appropriate for interpreting their results.[43] Time variables are included in three of the studies to reflect changes in input prices and technology.

The Geomet analysis of the New Jersey program involved the estimation of quasi-technological average-cost functions using data for New Jersey hospitals and for twenty-eight control hospitals in the eastern portion of Pennsylvania for the years 1968–1973.[44] Some cost regressions were also estimated on a subsample of twenty-eight New Jersey hospitals (in which quality of care was also studied) and the twenty-eight control hospitals, while still other regressions did not include the control hospitals. In most cases all six years of data were included, although some equations were estimated with data for single years or selected groups of years. Both linear and log-linear (double-log) functional forms were employed. The effect of the rate-setting program was represented by the coefficient of a single dummy variable indicating whether a hospital was subject to rate setting.[45]

While the Geomet researchers were most thorough in their testing of different regression specifications, presenting no less than fifty-eight estimates of the rate-setting coefficient, these estimates were both negative and greater than their estimated standard errors in only a few instances. One of these instances was the cost-per-case regression (using 1970–1973 data for New Jersey hospitals), which included the most complete specification of case-mix variables. Nevertheless, the omission of control hospitals from this regression, as well as the bulk of the other evidence presented, leads to the conclusion that the New Jersey program had no negative impact on average cost. A more hopeful result might have been obtained with a more complex specification of the rate-setting variables[46] and the availability of case-mix data for both experimental and control hospitals, but we have no evidence to support this conjecture.[47]

In Thornberry and Zimmerman's study of the Rhode Island program, linear and log-linear cost functions were estimated with 1969–1972 data, for all thirteen Rhode Island hospitals and with 1971–1972 data for the Rhode Island hospitals and twelve control hospitals in Massachusetts.[48] A dummy variable for Rhode Island hospitals in 1971–1972 was included to

Table 4-1
Hospital Cost Regression Models Used in the Five Rate-Setting Studies

	Indiana	New Jersey[a]	Downstate New York	Upstate New York	Rhode Island
Study period	1968–73	1968–73	1968–74	1968–74	1969–72
Control areas	Illinois, Iowa, Michigan, Minnesota	Southeastern Pennsylvania	Chicago, Cleveland, and Philadelphia SMSAs	Northern Ohio, Southeastern Michigan, and the Milwaukee SMSA	Massachusetts
Dependent variables	Average cost per admission	Average cost per day Average cost per admission	Average cost per day[b] Average cost per admission[b]	Total Cost[c] Average Cost per Day[c] Average Cost per Admission[c]	Average Cost per Day[d] Average Cost per Discharge[d]
Independent variables[e]	Average length of stay Interns and residents per bed Ratio of outpatient and emergency to total charges Ratio of ECF reds to total beds Number of the month ending the fiscal year Ratio of office-based physicians to population[i] Median 1969 family income[i] Percentage white population in 1970[i] Nonprofit hospital dummy Indiana hospital dummy	Average daily census Occupancy rate Caseflow rate Admissions per day Urban location dummy Rate setting dummy Dummy variable for first year under rate-setting (1970, 1971, 1972, 1973+) Individual year dummies (1969–73) Council of Teaching Hospitals member dummy Organized outpatient clinic dummy Two service-mix dummies (quality enhancing and community)[j]	Admissions Patient Days Beds Occupancy Rate AMA-Approved Residency Dummy Accreditation Status[g] Weighted Sum of Facilities and Services Offered[h] Time Trend for 1968–74 Time Trend for 1970–74 Dummy Variable for 1970–74 Observations	Admissions Patient Days Beds Occupancy Rate Average Length of Stay Facilities and Services Dummies (21) Individual Year Dummies (1966–74) 1965–69 Time Trend for Experimental Hospitals 1965–69 Time Trend for Control Hospitals 1970–74 Time Trend for Experimental Hospitals 1970–74 Time Trend for Control Hospitals	Average Length of Stay Occupancy Rate Beds Teaching Activity Index[f] Percentages of Patients in Each of 17 ICDA Groups Percentage of Patients Under 14 Percentage of Patients Over 65 Percentage of Patients with Surgery Rate Setting Dummy

1965–69 Dummy for Experimental Hospitals

1970–74 Dummy for Experimental Hospitals

1970–74 Dummy for Control Hospitals

1970 Population[1]

1970 Population Density[1]

1970 Per Cent Population Under 5[1]

1970 Per Cent Population 18–64[1]

1970 Per Cent Urban Population[1]

1969 Income per Capita[1]

Mean Disposable Family Income[1]

Per Cent of Population with 1969 Income Under 125% of Poverty Level[1]

Outpatient Visits

Per Cent of 1970 Workers in Construction[1]

Per Cent of 1970 Workers in Manufacturing[1]

Number of Hospital Beds[1]

Number of General Practitioners[1]

Number of Specialists[1]

[a]In addition to the independent variables listed, several other types of variables were used only occasionally in the regression analyses. These variables pertained to patient mix (based on ICDA codes), wage rate, staffing mix and intensity, service intensity, and quality of care (based on medical record audits).

[b]Adjusted for outpatient expense and deflated by a regional price index.

[c]This variable was used both with and without adjustment for outpatient expenses.

[d]Deflated by a regional index of hospital costs. Reported costs of outpatient services, research, and education are excluded.

[e]All variables used in the primary regression analyses of each study are listed here. However, all listed variables were not always included in the same regression equation. Other variables used in subsidiary or peripheral analyses and variables deleted from the primary regressions in some studies are not listed here.

[f]This index "assigns three points to a hospital for an approved residency program, two points for each approved internship or nursing program, and one point for the affiliation of a hospital with a teaching program." See Helen Thornberry and Harvey Zimmerman, *Hospital Cost Control: An Assessment of the Rhode Island Experience with Prospective Reimbursement, 1971 and 1972*, Final Report on Contract HEW-OS-74-197 (Providence, R.I.: Rhode Island Health Services Research, n.d.), p. 136.

[g]Unaccredited = 0, one-year (provisional) accreditation = 1, and two-year (full) accreditation = 2.

[h]Weights reflect expected costliness of each facility and service.

[i]This variable is defined for the county in which the hospital is located.

[j]Each hospital was assigned to either the quality-enhancing, community, or basic categories based on its facilities and services as reported in the American Hospital Association annual survey.

estimate the effect of rate setting. To control for exogenous inflationary trends, the dependent variables were deflated by regional hospital cost indexes. These indexes measured yearly increases in the average cost of a hospital day (or hospital stay), adjusted for changes in the relative importance of outpatient activity, in New England hospitals.

There are several important problems in the design of Thornberry and Zimmerman's analysis. First, the small number of data points (fifty or fifty-two) made it difficult to obtain accurate coefficient estimates, particularly since the regressions included approximately twenty explanatory variables. As a result, most of these variables—including ones that have been significant in previous studies, such as the occupancy rate—did not have significant coefficients. Second, the meaning of the rate-setting dummy's coefficient in the regressions with 1969–1972 data for Rhode Island hospitals is clouded by the lack of a control group. In particular, this coefficient may reflect the combined effects of the Rhode Island program and federal price controls (introduced in August 1971), though the use of a regional hospital cost index as a deflator mitigates this problem somewhat by controlling for regional trends. Third, the 1971–1972 regressions with both Rhode Island and Massachusetts hospitals are not very informative because of the lack of pre-rate-setting data. In particular, it is unclear whether the rate-setting coefficients in these regressions measure actual effects of rate-setting or existing differences in cost levels between the two states. All three of these problems would have been alleviated by estimating regressions with 1969–1972 data for both states.[49]

Estimated coefficients of the rate-setting dummy were consistently negative but were more significant in the cost-per-case regressions (t-values ranged from 1.6 to 2.7) than in those for cost per day (t-values ranged from 0.9 to 1.4). Rate-setting effects estimated from the 1969–1972 Rhode Island data were more significant than those based on 1971–1972 data for both states. The magnitudes of these coefficients implied that the Rhode Island program reduced hospital costs by 2 percent to 5 percent. Of course, this result cannot be viewed as conclusive because of the research design problems.[50]

An alternative procedure developed by Silverman yielded a smaller estimate of cost savings.[51] This procedure used 1969–1970 data for the same experimental and control hospitals to estimate cost functions.[52] The estimated coefficients were then used to predict 1971 and 1972 cost levels in the control hospitals, and the excess of their actual costs over the predictions was computed. The same procedure was carried out for the experimental (Rhode Island) hospitals with the result that the excess of actual over predicted costs was slightly less than for the control hospitals. Attributing this differential to the Rhode Island program, Silverman reported essentially no reduction in cost per day and a 2.2 percent saving in cost per case.

The analyses of the upstate and downstate New York programs are of special interest for several reasons. The general presumption that rates under these programs were stringently controlled leads one to expect clear evidence of cost savings. Since these analyses examined five years of experience with the programs (1970–1974), their results should be less distorted by an atypical start-up period or the confounding influence of federal price controls. The length of the study period and the large number of hospitals in each program minimize the possibility of estimation problems due to limited sample sizes.

The examination of the upstate program by Abt Associates was based on data for 63 experimental hospitals and 56 control-group hospitals (from Michigan, Ohio, and Wisconsin) for the years 1965–1974.[53] These hospitals were selected from the total of 265 hospitals in the study and control areas on the basis of data availability and the criteria that no more than 10 percent of their beds were in long-term care units. The size of Abt's data base made it possible to include a large number of explanatory variables in the regressions, including (in some regressions) a number of exogenous variables pertaining to the county in which a hospital was located. These variables were selected to control for variations in product demand.[54] No explanation is given, however, for the absence of variables relating to factor-supply conditions. The only exogenous demand variable that changes over time is income. Since the dependent variables are not deflated by a price index and factor-price variables are not included, and since the regressions with income also include linear time-trend variables, income presumably serves as a proxy for any inflationary influences not captured by these time-trend variables.

Results are reported for two linear regression models. The first model includes all the explanatory variables listed in table 4–1 except the individual year dummies. The specification of the rate-setting and time variables in this model corresponds to that of equation 4.4. In the second model only beds, occupancy rate, the teaching hospital dummy, outpatient visits, and the facilities and services dummies were used as explanatory variables. Dummy variables were also included for each of the years 1966–1974. The effect of rate setting was estimated by including dummy variables for experimental hospitals in the post-rate-setting years (1970–1974), for control hospitals in these same years, and for control hospitals in the pre-rate-setting years (1965–1969).[55] An important difference between these models is that the first permits the effect of rate-setting to vary over time while the second assumes that this effect is constant.

The first regression model may be more appealing because of its more general specification for rate-setting effects, but the procedures used by Abt to calculate these effects and their significance levels contain two technical errors. One of these errors results from defining the rate-setting effect solely in terms of the differential change in time-trend coefficients, or in the notation of equation 4.4, $(\gamma_4 - \gamma_3) - (\gamma_2 - \gamma_1)$. This formulation omits the differential shift in intercepts, $(\alpha_4 - \alpha_3) - (\alpha_2 - \alpha_1)$, which should also be attributed to rate setting. The second error occurs in computing the standard deviation of the estimate $(\hat{\gamma}_4 - \hat{\gamma}_3) - (\hat{\gamma}_2 - \hat{\gamma}_1)$. Based on the assertion that the covariances of the $\hat{\gamma}$'s are zero because they apply to mutually exclusive groups of hospitals, this standard deviation is calculated as $[\text{var}(\hat{\gamma}_1) + \text{var}(\hat{\gamma}_2) + \text{var}(\hat{\gamma}_3) + \text{var}(\hat{\gamma}_4)]^{1/2}$. But this is incorrect because the covariances of the $\hat{\gamma}$'s are not in general zero.[56] This second error probably recurs in Abt's computation of standard deviations for the rate-setting effects in their second model $[(\hat{\alpha}_4 - \hat{\alpha}_3) - (\hat{\alpha}_2 - \hat{\alpha}_1)]$ although their report is not explicit on this point.[57]

Abt's reported rate-setting effects for the first model $[(\hat{\gamma}_4 - \hat{\gamma}_3) - (\hat{\gamma}_2 - \hat{\gamma}_1)]$ are consistently negative for all dependent variables. However, when the omitted portion of these effects $[(\hat{\alpha}_4 - \hat{\alpha}_3) - (\hat{\alpha}_2 - \hat{\alpha}_1)]$ is considered, the picture is less clear. In the regressions of cost per patient-day this omitted portion is either negative or positive but of the same order of magnitude as the reported effect. In the cost-per-admission and total-cost regressions the omitted effect is generally positive and two to five times larger than the reported effect. It seems therefore likely that the correctly computed effects $[(\hat{\alpha}_4 - \hat{\alpha}_3) - (\hat{\alpha}_2 - \hat{\alpha}_1) + (\hat{\gamma}_4 - \hat{\gamma}_3)T - (\hat{\gamma}_2 - \hat{\gamma}_1)T]$ are more clearly and consistently negative for cost per day than for cost per case or total cost.[58]

A similar pattern is observed with Abt's second model. Rate-setting effects on cost per case are positive while the impacts on cost per day and total cost are negative when these dependent variables are adjusted for outpatient visits. (The effect on total cost is, however, very weak.) Without the outpatient adjustment, the effect on cost per day is virtually zero while the total cost impact is positive. Of course, the statistical significance of any of these effects is unclear because of the possibility of error in computing their standard deviations.

The downstate New York analysis, by Dowling and his associates, involved estimation of average-cost regressions for the 1968–1974 period with data from hospitals in southeastern New York and control groups from the three metropolitan areas of Chicago, Cleveland, and Philadelphia.[59] The dependent variables were adjusted for the volume of outpatient activity (measured by each hospital's ratio of outpatient to total revenues) and were deflated by a price index to control for inflation in input prices. The price index was a weighted average of indexes for a number of inputs, with wage increases accounting for roughly 60 percent of the index.

Separate indexes were calculated for downstate New York and for each of the three control regions. This deflation procedure is designed to control for inflation within each area rather than differences in input price levels across the four areas.[60]

As table 4–1 indicates, the quasi-technological type of cost function was employed in the study. For the most part, separate equations were estimated for each of the four areas, with a shift in the intercept and in the coefficient of the time trend specified for the post-rate-setting period (1970–1974).[61] Both linear and log-linear functional forms were used.[62]

As in the upstate New York study, the estimated impact of rate setting was defined as the difference in the post-rate setting shifts of the time-trend coefficients for the experimental and control groups. Thus the difference in intercept shifts was again incorrectly ignored. Differences in the shifts of time-trend coefficients between experimental hospitals and the Philadelphia and Cleveland control groups indicate reductions in cost due to rate setting but are not statistically significant. With the Chicago control group the surprising result of significant increases in costs due to rate setting is obtained. Moreover, shifts in intercepts are almost always more positive for experimental hospitals than for any of the control groups, casting further doubt on the possibility that the downstate New York program achieved significant cost savings.[63]

Oddly enough, other regressions referred to in the report that used only data from nonprofit hospitals indicated significantly negative differences in the shifts of time-trend coefficients between experimental hospitals and all control hospitals, implying that rate setting had reduced the rate of cost increase.[64] Data for all experimental and control hospitals in these other regressions were apparently combined.[65] Separate intercepts (both before and after rate setting) were allowed for each of the four areas while two sets of before and after time-trend coefficients were estimated (one for experimental hospitals and one for controls). Unfortunately, the full results of these regressions were not reported, so the signs and magnitudes of the differences in intercept shifts cannot be determined.[66]

Other regressions indicating significant cost savings are reported by Hellinger in his review of the downstate New York study.[67] These regressions are log-linear in form, and data for all four areas for the 1968–1973 period are included in each. Two separate intercepts (one for experimental and one for control hospitals) are specified, and dummy variables for the years 1970–1973 rather than a linear time trend are included. The effect of rate setting is estimated by including a single rate-setting dummy (equal to one for experimental hospitals in the years 1970–1973). The coefficients for this dummy are significantly negative, indicating that rate setting reduced cost per day by about 5 percent and cost per case by about

8.5 percent. However, several curious aspects of these regressions diminish confidence in the reported findings. For example, no explanation is given for the exclusion of 1974 data from the analysis or the failure to include a dummy variable for the year 1969. Similarly, no justification is given for the restrictive assumption (implied by the regression specification) that the rate-setting effect is constant in percentage terms over time. In view of these limitations and the rather mixed findings presented in the report of the downstate New York study, Hellinger's conclusion that the downstate New York program reduced costs does not have a very firm basis.[68]

Because the Indiana program has been in operation since 1960, analysis with a before-and-after design would present some difficulties. A consistent and substantial data base would be difficult to obtain because of changes in the availability and definitions of specific items of data. The structural changes in the health system during the 1960s and early 1970s, such as the advent of Medicare and Medicaid and the expansion of internship and residency programs, make it unlikely that hospital cost behavior in this period could be adequately described by a single set of regression coefficients. The Indiana study by Spectrum Research therefore relied instead on cost comparisons between Indiana and control hospitals during the 1968–1973 period.[69] Although these comparisons do not measure the total effect of rate-setting, they can at least indicate whether costs rose more or less rapidly (in absolute or relative terms) in Indiana during this period.[70]

Two groups of control hospitals were used in the Indiana study. One was selected from three nearby states lacking in regulatory controls during the study period (Illinois, Iowa, and Minnesota), while the other was selected from a nearby state in which Blue Cross reviewed proposed capital expansion projects (Michigan).[71] Since Indiana Blue Cross also reviewed capital expenditure proposals, cost comparisons between Indiana and Michigan hospitals were intended to measure the incremental effect of rate setting when investment controls are already in place. However, Spectrum's use of cost regressions based solely on Indiana and Michigan data, with an Indiana dummy variable included to measure this incremental effect, raises a question of interpretation. The specification of these regressions was based on a model of individual hospital behavior, and the rate-setting variable was included to measure the deviation of actual costs from the cost levels to be expected if the behavior of Indiana hospitals was in accordance with this model and free from regulatory constraints.[72] But when the control-group hospitals are themselves subject to regulatory constraints, this interpretation is not strictly correct. In such an instance it would be preferable to develop the regression specification from a conceptual model that describes the behavior of both hospitals and regulators in the control state.[73] An alternative approach, not requiring a new conceptual model, is to use an additional control group from a state with no regulation and to include additional regulatory variables for hospitals in the original control group.[74]

The Spectrum report presents three sets of linear regression equations. One set analyzes data for Indiana and the Illinois-Iowa-Minnesota control group, a second is based on Indiana and Michigan data, and a third uses data for Indiana and both control groups. Within each set single-year cross-sectional regressions are estimated for 1968, 1970, 1972, and 1973, and a cross-sectional percentage change regression is estimated for the 1968–1973 period. In all regressions a dummy variable for Indiana hospitals is included.

Results for the single-year regressions indicate a time trend of increasingly negative and significant coefficients for the Indiana dummy, suggesting that the Indiana program did indeed reduce the rate of cost increase. This is further corroborated by findings from the percentage change regressions. More specifically, Spectrum's estimates indicate that the percentage cost increase from 1968 to 1973 was one-tenth to one-fifth lower in Indiana hospitals because of rate setting.

Despite this clear evidence that the Indiana program succeeded in holding down the rate of cost increases, it may be prudent to view this conclusion as tentative because of several debatable features of the regression analyses. In particular, the reported single-year regressions include only the small number of explanatory variables whose coefficients were highly (95 percent) significant. As a result, such commonly used variables as bed size, insurance coverage, and the urban or rural nature of the hospital's location do not appear. Moreover, because the dependent variables are not deflated and no factor-price or wage variables are included, differences in results between the 1968 and 1973 regressions may be partially due to differing inflation rates in Indiana and neighboring states.[75] Similarly, the failure to include changes in income levels and factor prices or wages in the percentage change regressions is also disturbing. Admittedly, there is no particular reason to believe that inclusion of these variables would radically alter Spectrum's results, but empirical evidence to the contrary would make their results more definitive.

Finally, Spectrum also presents a simple comparison of trends in average cost per case that supports their econometric results. Average cost per case in Indiana hospitals was 5 percent below that of control hospitals in 1958, 1959, and 1960. But by 1976 this differential widened to 17 percent. On the other hand, results are not quite so clear when Indiana is compared with each of the four control states. For example, American Hospital Association *Guide Issue* data show a 332 percent increase in cost per case of Indiana hospitals over the 1960–1975 period. This is lower than the increases of 343 percent and 395 percent for Illinois and Michigan respectively but greater than Iowa's 320 percent increase or the 296 percent increase for Minnesota. Similarly, *Guide Issue* data indicate that the 1960–1975 relative increase in average cost per day for Indiana (323 percent) is again less than the increases for Illinois (357 percent) and Michigan (349 percent) but greater than the corresponding figures for Iowa (304 percent) and Minnesota (259 percent).[76] The results of these comparisons at least raise the possibility that the estimated impact of the Indiana program is sensitive to the choice of the control group.[77]

In attempting to assess and interpret the results of these five studies, one should consider several methodological issues common to most or all of these studies. In particular, the appropriateness of relying solely on the simple ordinary least-squares estimation techniques is unclear when pooled data are used and in view of possible simultaneity bias. Reestimation of some of the regression models with methods developed for the analysis of pooled data and with two-stage least squares (in the case of the quasi-technological cost functions) would therefore have been of particular interest.[78] Another limitation of these studies, resulting from the use of the individual hospital as the unit of analysis, is the omission of cost impacts arising from program effects on the opening of new hospitals and the closing or merging of old ones. These impacts could have been captured through the estimation of total-cost regressions with data aggregated over geographical areas, although this aggregation would entail a loss of information in the estimation process. Furthermore, results obtained with average cost (per day or per case) as the dependent variable cannot be translated into estimated impacts on total hospital costs without an examination of program impacts on the volume of services. Finally, even the estimated average-cost impacts may be incomplete measures of actual rate-setting effects on average costs because of the importance in the regressions of explanatory variables such as length of stay and the occupancy rate, which are themselves likely to be influenced by rate setting. In view of these last two limitations, it is important to consider evidence from these studies of rate-setting effects on admissions rates, length of stay, and occupancy rates.

Other Types of Program Impacts

Evidence, from four of the five studies, of rate-setting impacts on admissions, length of stay, case-mix, occupancy rates, patient days, outpatient visits, capital stock, and scope of services,[79] when viewed in conjunction with the average cost analyses, permits some tentative conclusions about the impact of rate-setting on total hospital costs. Then impacts on quality and financial position are reviewed.[80]

Judgments about the Rhode Island program's effects are highly tentative because they are based on comparisons of trend data covering a very short time period.[81] Average length of stay declined in Rhode Island hospitals from 1969 to 1971 but then increased in 1972 while a steady decline was observed in Massachusetts control hospitals over the 1969–1972 period. To the extent that the reversal in trend in Rhode Island was due to rate setting, it offsets the negative effect of rate setting on average cost per case, since length of stay was significantly positive in the regressions of average cost per case.

Comparisons of trends in bed complements and occupancy rates do not provide even suggestive evidence of rate-setting effects. Average beds increased steadily in both Rhode Island hospitals and control hospitals. The average occupancy rate increased in Rhode Island hospitals from 1969 to 1970 and then fluctuated while it declined steadily in control hospitals. A comparison of changes in the costliness of case mix between 1970 and 1972 (using case-mix coefficients from Silverman's cost functions based on 1969 and 1970 data) shows more of a shift toward a less costly case mix in Rhode Island than in control hospitals when the unit of analysis is the patient-day, but this differential shift is minimal on a per case basis.[82]

In summary, the apparent lack of rate-setting effects in these trend comparisons gives little reason to suspect substantial program impacts on total costs. Similarly, the possible effects on length of stay and case mix have offsetting cost implications. Since the Rhode Island cost analysis indicated that rate setting had lowered average cost per day and per case by only a very small amount, it appears that the negative impact on total hospital costs was probably minimal.

Abt's analysis of the upstate New York program presents comparisons of experimental and control hospitals for bed complement, length of stay, occupancy rate, admissions, patient-days, and outpatient visits.[83] Inspection of trends over the 1965–1974 period indicates that both beds and admissions increased somewhat more rapidly in control hospitals, although this difference was already observable in 1968 and thus may not be attributable to the implementation of rate setting in 1970. Conversely, outpatient visits increased more rapidly in experimental hospitals over the entire ten-year period, while the trends in patient days were similar for both groups. Occupancy rates rose more rapidly in experimental hospitals from 1965 to 1968 and then declined in both groups. Trends in average length of stay were also similar in both groups except for a sharp increase in experimental hospitals from 1972 to 1974. This increase may have been due to the introduction into the rate-setting program in 1971 of penalties for hospitals falling below minimum occupancy rates.

The Abt report also refers to estimated rate-setting effects on these same variables that are "net of the exogenous variables" (p. V-46). Presumably these estimates are obtained from regression analyses similar to those used in estimating cost impacts, although no mention or description of such analyses is contained in the report. In contrast to the trend comparisons, these estimates show negative effects of rate setting on patient-days, occupancy, length of stay, and outpatient visits. Estimated effects on bed size and admissions are reported to be negligible.[84]

Analyses of wage levels and scope of services and facilities were also included in the upstate New York study (in chapters 8 and 11 respectively). Both trend comparisons and multivariate analyses of wages (average hospital salaries) failed to reveal any perceptible rate-setting effect. In the scope-of-service analysis selected facilities and services reported in the American Hospital Association annual surveys were divided into three groups: quality enhancing, complexity expanding, and community services.[85] The number of services in each of the three groups reported by each hospital was computed for the years 1969–1974. Multiple regression analyses of the yearly percentage change in each of these three indicators were then carried out with data from both experimental and control hospitals. Rate-setting effects were estimated by including separate intercept and time-trend variables for experimental hospitals. The coefficients of these variables were small and insignificant except for the time-trend variable in the complexity-expanding regression. Moreover, the rate-setting intercept in this regression was also large but positive and nearly significant ($t = 1.4$). A joint test of these two coefficients would presumably fail to show a significantly negative rate-setting effect.[86] On the other hand, simple comparisons of the percentage changes in the three scope-of-service indicators from 1969 to 1974 for each of three hospital size groups (100 beds, 100–300 beds, and 300+ beds) indicate smaller increases in complexity-expanding services for experimental hospitals. Comparisons of percentages of hospitals with each of thirty-two specific facilities or services in 1969 and 1974 (chapter 10 of the Abt report) also support this finding. Percentages of hospitals with cardiac care units, open heart surgery, therapeutic radiology services, and several other specialized facilities increased more rapidly or decreased less rapidly in the control groups, although this was not true for several other services.

To assess the implications for average costs of these rate-setting effects, the Abt report (chapter 5) compares cost regressions that include beds, admissions, length of stay, occupancy, patient-days, and facilities and services dummies as explanatory variables with regressions that exclude these variables. The similarity of estimated rate-setting effects on costs implies that rate-setting impacts on these explanatory variables had little influence on average cost levels. Little can be said about possible total-cost implications of rate-setting effects on admissions, beds, patient-days, and outpatient visits because the Abt analysis included only about one-third of all the hospitals in the experimental and control regions.

The downstate New York study presents trend comparisons over the 1968–1974 period (chapter 4) for length of stay, scope of services, occupancy rates, wages, and for admissions per capita in the control and experimental areas. The last figure was stable in both areas before rate setting (1968 and 1969) and then increased more rapidly in downstate New York (16.5 percent) than in the control area (9.0 percent) from 1969 to 1974. Length of stay was declining for experimental hospitals and stable for control hospitals during 1968 and 1969 but then declined more rapidly in control hospitals (2.2 percent yearly) than in experimental hospitals (1.0 percent yearly). Occupancy comparisons for nonprofit hospitals show a slow and steady increase for experimental hospitals and a decline for controls after 1970. The pattern for proprietary hospitals is similar, although the pre-rate-setting increase for experimental hospitals and the post-rate-setting decrease for controls were smaller (in percentage terms) than they were for the voluntaries.

To measure scope of services, the presence or absence in each hospital of each of twenty-four facilities and services (reported in the American Hospital Association's annual surveys) during 1969–1974 was ascertained. Each facility and service offered was then multiplied by a costliness weight (assigned by panels of administrators and physicians), and these values were summed over all facilities and services offered by the hospital to obtain a scope-of-service indicator. Examination of this variable for the 1969–1974 period revealed the unexpected result that the scope of services was increasing more rapidly in downstate New York than in control hospitals. Finally, comparisons of wage (average salary) trends showed more rapid increases in downstate New York both before and after rate setting, though a different result might have been obtained if area differences in general inflation had been taken into account.[87]

These comparisons suggest that rate setting tended to increase the volume of inpatient care (admissions, length of stay, and patient-days) in the downstate New York area. Such an increase offsets cost savings from lower average costs due to the rate-setting program.[88] However, because the pre-rate-setting period examined in the study was only two years long, the trend-comparison evidence of rate-setting effects is not very compelling.[89]

Spectrum's study of the Indiana program presents regression analyses of case-flow rates, case mix, length of stay, wage levels, and capital stock variables using the same study designs employed in their cost analysis. Cross-sectional case-flow equations for the years 1968, 1970, 1972, and 1973 (chapter 23) show positive and sometimes significant coefficients for the Indiana dummy variable but no trend over these years. Similarly, the Indiana dummy is insignificant in the 1968–1973 percentage change formulation. Length of stay is an important predictor in all these regressions, so an indirect effect of the Indiana program (through its influence on length of stay) seems possible. In fact, cross-sectional regressions for 1970 and 1973 using three length-of-stay measures (chapter 30) generally show positive but not highly significant coefficients for the Indiana dummy variable.[90] However no upward trend from 1970 to 1973 is observed in these coefficients, and the coefficient of the Indiana dummy is insignificant and often negative in 1970–1973 percentage change regressions. Similar findings are obtained when a case-mix–costliness index is used as the dependent variable.

Two dependent variables were used in the wage analysis: average salary (chapter 23) and an index of nursing personnel wages (chapter 26). With the former the Indiana program was estimated to have a negative impact on wage increases over the 1968–1973 period when Michigan hospitals were the control group but an insignificantly positive impact with the Illinois-Iowa-Minnesota control group. For the latter dependent variable an insignificantly negative effect on wage increases was obtained with both control groups. However, explanatory power in all these regressions was low, perhaps because explanatory variables relating to labor-market conditions (such as wage levels outside the hospital sector) are not included.

Five investment measures were used in the Indiana study: change in assets per bed, change in beds, changes in two scope-of-service indexes (one for specialized and one for basic services), and investment spending over the 1968–1973 period. However, the regressions in which these measures were dependent variables generally showed no significant effects of the Indiana program.[91] The only exceptions were a negative effect on change in assets per bed over the 1968–1973 period with the Michigan control group and a positive effect on change in beds over this same period with the Michigan control group and with both control groups combined. The lack of significant results may, of course, be partly due to the restricted number of explanatory variables employed. Variables relating to availability of funds and to changes in demand conditions, which have been important in other studies of hospital investment,[92] were not included in Spectrum's reported regressions.

In short, the Spectrum report shows little evidence of rate-setting impacts on utilization, wage, and investment variables over the 1968–1973 period. But since the period covered by the report is brief relative to the

Table 4–2
Changes in Utilization for Indiana and the Control States
(in percent)

State	Admissions per Capita		Average Length of Stay		Inpatient Days per Capita	
	1960– 1975	*1965– 1975*	*1960– 1975*	*1965– 1975*	*1960– 1975*	*1965– 1975*
Indiana	33.5	19.0	2.6	−3.7	37.0	14.6
Illinois	26.1	15.7	−2.4	1.3	23.1	17.2
Iowa	37.0	19.9	2.6	−2.5	40.6	16.9
Michigan	17.0	19.9	9.3	2.5	27.9	22.9
Minnesota	10.9	6.8	10.0	12.8	22.0	20.5

Source: Computed from data in the 1961 and 1966 American Hospital Association *Guide Issues; Hospital Statistics,* 1978 edition (Chicago: American Hospital Association); and the *Statistical Abstract of the United States* (Washington, D.C.: U.S. Department of Commerce, various years).

Note: Data pertain to nonfederal short-term general and other special hospitals.

period of the Indiana program's operations, some simple comparisons of Indiana and the control states for the period 1960–1975 based on *Guide Issue* data may be of interest. These comparisons, which are shown in table 4–2 reveal relatively large increases in admissions per capita and patient-days per capita for Indiana in comparison with the control states and relatively small increases in average length of stay. On the other hand, in the 1965–1975 period the Indiana increases in admissions and inpatient-days per capita are not relatively large. This at least suggests that if rate setting had any positive effects on the volume of inpatient care, they occurred primarily in the early years of the Indiana program.

Several kinds of information were used to examine impacts on quality of care in the five studies. The New York studies relied primarily on opinions expressed by administrators and health professionals in the experimental hospitals, although the accuracy of these judgments is obviously open to question because they may reflect respondents' general like or dislike of the rate-setting program. Of more interest was the finding in the downstate New York study (chapter 4) that the percentage of hospitals receiving only provisional (one-year) approvals from the Joint Commission on Accreditation of Hospitals increased much more rapidly in the experimental group than in the control group over the 1968–1974 period.[93]

In the Indiana and New Jersey studies the content of care rendered to hospital patients (as indicated in medical records or record abstracts) was examined to determine quality impacts. Quality scores were assigned to each hospital based on the agreement between the care actually rendered and criteria determined by clinical experts. The Indiana study (chapters 29 and 31) constructed these scores from data on patients in fifteen different diagnostic groups for the years 1970 and 1973. Regression analysis of variations in these scores revealed no perceptible effect of the Indiana program. The New Jersey study (chapter 3) employed data on three diagnostic groups for the 1968–1973 period and again found no effect of rate setting. Finally, the Rhode Island study examined record-abstract data to determine percentages of patients not receiving certain basic diagnostic and laboratory services. These percentages did not generally increase for Rhode Island hospital's during the 1970–1972 rate-setting period; however, comparisons with control hospitals were not presented.

The dependent variables used in most of the analyses of financial impacts were measures of net revenue or profitability.[94] Spectrum's regression analysis of the Indiana program (chapter 27) showed significantly negative rate-setting effects on the 1973 ratio of net to total revenues and a significantly negative effect on the 1968–1973 change in this ratio. However, evidence of negative program effects on working capital was much weaker and not statistically significant. In the Rhode Island study (chapter 5) the profitability of experimental hospitals fluctuated during the period before rate setting (1968–1969), improved during the 1971 and 1972 rate-setting years, and then declined with the advent of Economic Stabilization Program (ESP) controls (1973). Comparable data for control hospitals were not reported. In the upstate New York study (chapter 5) 1968–1973 trend comparisons of net revenue per day showed erratic movements from 1968 to 1970 but a marked decline for experimental hospitals after 1970 in contrast to an increase for control hospitals. However, similar comparisons of the ratio of net to total revenue show a sharply declining trend for experimental hospitals even before 1970, suggesting that factors other than rate setting were adversely affecting their financial position. Abt's regression analysis of net revenue per day using 1965–1973 data showed a clearly negative rate-setting effect.[95]

The most detailed analysis of financial impacts was carried out by Dowling and his associates in the downstate New York study (chapter 7). Trends in ratios of net to total revenues, liquidity measures, debt measures, and the ratio of unrestricted endowment to total assets were compared for experimental and control hospitals over the years 1968–1974. Although net revenues were considerably more negative for experimental hospitals throughout the entire period, a trend toward more negative net to total revenue ratios was observed only for the control hospitals. On the other hand, the liquidity ratios (the current, quick, and acid test ratios) declined steadily for experimental hospitals but were fairly stable for controls.[96] Ratios of short-term debt to current liabilities, long-term debt to total assets, and total debt to total assets showed little or no evidence that rate setting increased reliance on debt financing. Finally, the ratio of unrestricted endowment funds to total assets declined precipitously in downstate New York voluntary hospitals, especially in the 1971–1974 period. For the control hospitals this ratio rose rapidly from 1968 to 1970, declined sharply in 1971, and then leveled off. Thus there is at least some evidence that hospitals responded to the financial pressures of the downstate New York program by eating into their endowment capital.[97]

Summary

Any attempt to review several thousand pages of material in a single brief essay is a perilous venture. Many facets of methods and research findings must be overlooked even though this runs the risk of leaving the reader with misinterpretations or false impressions. Nevertheless, on the presumption that fair warning has now been given, I shall proceed to compound this risk by restating in only a few paragraphs the major features of the results reviewed thus far.

Evidence of a negative rate-setting effect on average unit cost is generally meager, being weakest in the New Jersey and upstate New York studies and somewhat stronger in the Indiana study. Moreover, the cost savings found in Indiana and in some of the downstate New York analyses appear to be somewhat sensitive to the control groups and regression models employed. Of course, technical problems in some of the five studies and the brevity of most of the study periods may help to account for the statistically insignificant findings.[98]

Furthermore, there is fragmentary evidence that the volume of inpatient services was increased under rate setting. In particular, the behavior of length of stay in Rhode Island and both New York programs and the trends in admissions and patient-days per capita in the first five years of the Indiana program support this view. (But the subsequent Indiana experience suggests that this response to rate setting may be transient.) Such an increase in volume, which seems consistent with incentives under rate-setting programs, would tend to increase total cost and thus offset savings from lower unit costs. However, the evidence of volume increases is even weaker than that for reductions in unit costs.

Negative rate-setting effects on investment and financial position indicate the likelihood of future cost savings. But essentially no impacts on investment were found, with the possible exception of the scope-of-service analysis in upstate New York. The case for negative effects on profitability and other financial measures is stronger, particularly in the Indiana and upstate and downstate New York analyses.

Finally, the fairly detailed work on quality of care in New Jersey and

Indiana shows no adverse rate-setting impacts. Little hard evidence for quality impairment is found in the other studies, although the downstate New York data on provisional accreditations point in this direction.

Econometric Studies of Federal Price Controls

Direct federal intervention to control hospital cost inflation, as well as inflation in other sectors of the economy, began with Phase I of the Economic Stabilization Program (ESP), a ninety-day wage and price freeze from August 15 to November 14, 1971.[99] During this period hospitals were not permitted to increase either room charges or their specific service charges. However, neither the total cost of hospital care nor average cost per day (or per case) was directly constrained since increases in admissions, patient-days, length of stay, and the volume of ancillary services were not restricted. Furthermore, the freeze on prices did not clearly apply to the majority of hospital revenues, which were obtained directly from third parties through cost reimbursement.

Phase II ESP regulations for hospitals were issued December 30, 1971.[100] These regulations limited the annual rate of wage increases to 5.5 percent and stipulated that annual increases in total revenues due to price increases should not exceed 6 percent.[101] Reimbursements of costs from third parties were specifically included under this revenue limitation. The regulations did not, however, specify procedures for determining either total revenue increases due to price increases or the base-period figure against which such increases would be compared.

In an effort to clarify the situation, the Price Commission (which administered the ESP program) subsequently fixed January 1, 1971, as the date for determining base-period prices. However, this rule was difficult to apply to third-party cost reimbursements, since they were determined for an entire fiscal year rather than for each date within the year. Rulings issued in July and September of 1972 changed the base period for both revenues and costs to the hospital's last completed fiscal year.

To determine revenue increases due to price increases, it is necessary to compute the change in the volume of services from the base period. Procedures for this computation were not determined by the Price Commission until September 1972. The volume index promulgated at that time was a weighted combination of changes in admissions, inpatient-days, and outpatient procedures plus a 2 percent factor to reflect increases in service intensity. To correct technical errors in the formulation of this index, the Price Commission issued a revised formula in April 1973.[102]

As a result of the apparent stringency of Phase II controls and the delays and confusion relating to specific regulations, a large number of hospitals requested exceptions. These were first reviewed by advisory boards in each state that made recommendations to the Price Commission. The commission was responsible for rendering final decisions on each case but in practice delegated some of these decisions to the Internal Revenue Service. Specific guidelines for these decisions were not defined, but one general policy that emerged was the granting of exceptions necessary to avoid negative cash flows that would have resulted from strict adherence to controls.

Since not all hospitals were required to report financial data to the Price Commission, limited spot-checks of nonreporting hospitals were carried out by the Internal Revenue Service. However, the ambiguities in the program up to September 1972 made it difficult to determine whether hospitals were in compliance.

Another major deficiency in the ESP procedures was the failure to recognize the difference between average and marginal costs. In view of the empirical evidence that average costs exceed marginal costs (at least in the short run),[103] the volume index used in the program created strong incentives for hospitals to expand the numbers of admissions, patient-days, and outpatient visits. This problem was corrected by a new set of regulations drawn up for Phase IV of the program,[104] but these were never implemented since the ESP was terminated April 30, 1974.[105]

The behavior of several widely used indicators of hospital cost inflation during the period of the ESP indicates that the program was indeed successful in controlling costs. As table 4–3 shows, the rate of increase in cost per day (in constant dollars) declined sharply from 1972 to 1974. This was due to a decline in the rates of growth of both real average salaries and input quantities used to produce a day of care. On the other hand, an increased rate of growth in the volume of hospital services also occurred in the 1972–1974 period. This resulted from increases in admissions and a slackening of the decline in average length of stay. This increased volume may have been partly the result of the ESP program's failure to distinguish between average and marginal cost. Of course, to more rigorously assess the effects of the ESP, one must account for other factors that influenced the behavior of hospital costs during the ESP period, by means of a multiple regression analysis. Five recent studies used this approach.

Ginsburg employed quarterly data on the nine census divisions for the years 1963–1973 to estimate regressions in which the dependent variables included measures of utilization (such as admissions, patient-days, average length of stay, and outpatient visits), measures of average cost and average input use (per day and per case adjusted for outpatient visits), and average salaries.[106] Using the behavioral approach to specify the regression model, he included explanatory variables relating to general wage

Table 4–3
Annual Changes in Hospital Costs, Inputs, Salaries, and Utilization
(in percent)

	1969–1970	1970–1071	1971–1972	1972–1973	1973–1974	1974–1975
Average cost per day (in constant dollars)	9.2	9.2	10.3	2.6	0.6	8.4
Inputs per day	6.7	5.6	7.2	3.6	3.8	7.4
Average salary (in constant dollars)	4.0	5.8	4.6	−1.5	−4.9	1.6
Inpatient days	1.7	0.5	−0.1	2.6	2.9	1.0
Admissions	3.5	3.0	2.1	3.2	3.7	1.7
Average length of stay	−1.2	−2.4	−1.3	−1.3	0.0	−1.3

Sources: Rows 1–3, Martin Feldstein and Amy Taylor, "The Rapid Rise of Hospital Costs," Harvard Institute of Economic Research Discussion Paper 531, Cambridge, Mass., January 1977. Rows 4–6, *Hospital Statistics,* 1978 edition (Chicago: American Hospital Association), table 1.

Note: Data pertain to nonfederal short-term general and other special hospitals.

and price inflation, insurance coverage, population characteristics, and other factors presumed to be exogenous to the hospital. The impact of the ESP was accounted for by including a dummy variable equal to one when the program was in effect.

Results from Ginsburg's estimated regressions showed strongly negative ESP effects on salaries, average costs per case, patient-days, and average length of stay. However, since the negative effect on average length of stay contradicted the a priori expectation that incentives created by the ESP program would cause longer hospital stays, it was viewed as spurious and the regressions were reestimated with average length of stay included as an explanatory variable.[107] In this case the effects of ESP on wages, admissions, and patient-days were significantly negative, but the effect on average cost per case was not. In both sets of regressions average per diem cost was not affected by the ESP. Similar results were also obtained in regression models with a lagged dependent variable and models with the dependent variable in first-difference form.

Sloan and Steinwald used annual data for the 1970–1975 period on a national sample of 1,228 hospitals to estimate the effects of a variety of regulatory programs. Their dependent variables included average cost per day (adjusted for outpatient visits) and per admission, labor expense per day and per admission, ratios of employees (RNs, LPNs, and others) to beds, assets per bed, and total beds.[108] Explanatory variables pertained to product-demand and factor-supply conditions, regulation, and hospital characteristics (type of ownership, size, and teaching status).[109] Regressions with and without lagged dependent variables were estimated.[110]

In the regressions with lagged dependent variables, the ESP program had significantly negative effects on cost per day and per case but significantly positive effects on labor cost per day and per case. In regressions without lagged dependent variables only the positive effects on labor cost per day and per case were significant; effects on cost per day and per case were insignificantly positive. Negative effects on the employee per bed ratio and assets per bed were also observed, though these were only significant in half of the reported regressions.

Since these studies were carefully designed and executed, the presence of anomalous results is puzzling. Ginsburg's finding of a negative effect on wages and little effect on costs seems to imply a positive effect on inputs per day or per case. However, ESP coefficients in the input regressions were not significantly positive. Moreover, the significantly negative effect on length of stay was contrary to expectations. Sloan and Steinwald's findings of significantly negative effects on average costs and significantly positive effects on average labor costs are also difficult to reconcile. The authors suggest that rising wages during the ESP years may explain this situation, but it is not clear why the ESP program should have caused wages to rise.[111] Moreover, Ginsburg's results contradict this explanation. Finally, the difference in results between the two studies is not too surprising in view of their methodological differences. Each covered a slightly different time period and used differing units of analysis, estimation techniques, and explanatory variables.[112] Nevertheless, the fact that these methodological details appear to have affected the findings indicates that ESP cost impacts were not overwhelming.

A third study presenting estimates of behavioral cost-determination models is the recent work by Salkever and Bice.[113] This study used pooled state data for the years 1968–1972 to estimate regressions with total hospital cost per capita, cost per inpatient-day, and days per capita as the dependent variables. Dummy variables for each year were included among the regressors, and the year-to-year differences in the dummy variable coefficients in the cost regressions measured inflationary forces not captured by other variables in the regressions. If the ESP program constrained costs, this would be indicated by a decline in these differences for 1971 and 1972.

In fact, some of the reported regressions of total cost per capita did show a marked decline in year-to-year differences for 1971 and 1972, though much of this was due to the estimated negative effect on patient-days per capita. (As in Ginsburg's study, one may question whether this negative utilization effect was actually due to ESP controls.) However, in other regressions, which included separate intercept terms for each state to control for omitted state-specific effects, no decline in year-to-year coefficient differences could be discerned.

Feldstein presents estimates of a three-equation behavioral model of hospital cost determination based on state data for the years 1959–1973.[114] The first two equations in this model are demand functions for hospital admissions and for length of stay. Together these functions determine the demand for days of inpatient care. It is also assumed that year-to-year increases in hospital prices and average costs are proportional to the "excess demand" for care, where excess demand is defined as the days of care demanded minus the product of the hospital's desired occupancy rate and its available bed-days. The price-adjustment equation, which represents this relationship, is the third equation of the model.

The effect of the ESP is estimated by including dummy variables for 1971, 1972, and 1973 in the price-adjustment regression. None of the dummy variable coefficients is negative, however, implying that the program did not reduce the rate of price inflation.

Evidence of ESP impacts based on a quasi-technological approach to modeling hospital costs is presented by Lave and Lave.[115] In particular, they base their work on a model in which a hospital's average cost is a function of its case mix, occupancy rate, bed size, teaching activities, and factor prices. Although case-mix variables are not available for their regressions, they present several approaches to circumvent this problem. Assuming that the case mix of each hospital does not change very much except in the long run, they employed pooled data on individual hospitals for the years 1964–1973 to estimate regressions in which the dependent and independent variables are defined in relative terms. In one specification each variable is defined as the value for a particular year divided by the mean value of the variable for the hospital over the entire period. In a second specification each variable is defined as an annual percentage change.[116]

Regressions were estimated for a national sample of 507 hospitals. Separate intercepts were included for each year in the study, and the estimated values for these intercepts may be used to examine the hypothesis that the ESP program reduced the rate of cost inflation during 1971–1973. The regression results indicate that the annual rate of cost increases during the 1968–1973 period fell by about 50 percent. Though this decline began during the 1968–1970 period, it clearly accelerated during the ESP years. This may be partly due to a decline in general inflation (as measured by increases in the CPI) during 1970–1972, but the rate of general inflation increased markedly in 1973. On the whole, then, the Lave and

Lave findings suggest that ESP controls did in fact reduce the rate of hospital cost inflation.

In conclusion, there is not much agreement among these five studies about the effectiveness of the ESP, though somewhat more support is found for the view that the rate of hospital inflation was reduced than for the finding of no effect. Furthermore, as was true for the programs reviewed in the second section of this chapter, the possibility that average cost savings were partially offset by increases in the volume of care cannot be dismissed. Of course, the lack of clear program impacts may relate to the very short period during which controls were operative. Only the study by Sloan and Steinwald, which included 1974 data, showed fairly strong evidence of cost savings except in the labor cost analysis, perhaps because of strong program impacts during late 1973 and early 1974.[117] One might conjecture that the other studies would have tended more toward this conclusion if they too had employed 1974 data.[118]

Conclusions and Future Research Directions

In spite of differences in data and methods, the studies reviewed have generally led to the conclusion that rate-setting programs did not dramatically affect the level of hospital costs. Several reasons can be advanced to explain this conclusion. To begin with, the operational histories of these programs were rather brief. Most had less than five years of experience during the periods covered by the evaluative studies. Given that their effects might not be felt immediately because of start-up problems and lags in hospital responses aimed at cutting costs, it is not surprising that the evidence of cost savings was quite meager, and it is possible that their longer-run effects on costs would be more substantial. Moreover, there is some empirical support for this view. Accounts of program operations reveal important changes in procedures during the study periods.[119] Furthermore, note that the strongest evidence of cost savings came from Indiana, the state that had the program with the longest history. The sporadic evidence of negative program effects on financial variables, such as net revenue and endowment, also supports the expectation of greater cost savings subsequent to the study periods.

Another explanation for the apparent lack of substantial cost savings is based on the research designs. As a statistical matter, it may be difficult to measure rate-setting effects when either the pre-rate-setting or post-rate-setting portions of the study period cover only a few years.[120] Although this difficulty could be remedied by using longer study periods, other fundamental structural changes in the health sector are more likely to occur over a longer period, thereby complicating the task of specifying appropriate statistical models.

More skeptical observers may explain the lack of success in controlling costs as confirmation of recent theories of regulatory behavior. For example, the capture theory suggests that regulators will become more concerned with the growth and financial well-being of the hospitals and their employees than with the public's interest in controlling costs.[121] Similarly, the political-economy theory indicates that regulators' efforts to control costs will be hampered by the difficulties of obtaining information necessary to the task, limitations on agency resources, and political and economic incentives that discourage stringent controls.[122] However, descriptions of rate-setting programs often reveal indications of regulators' strong interest in controlling costs and numerous examples of conflict with the regulated hospitals, particularly in the New York and ESP programs. Such behavior is not consistent with the capture and political-economy theories and warns that these theories may only be accurate in particular instances.[123]

The lack of cost impacts might also be explained with reference to hospital incentives. Although a rate-setting program can create a short-run incentive to cut costs and thereby generate positive net revenues, several factors tend to counteract this incentive.[124] One is that hospitals may be severely constrained in their use of these net revenues to finance new programs by rate-setting or planning authorities. Thus the accumulation of substantial net revenues may be of little value to the hospital (especially the nonprofit hospital). When current cost levels serve as a basis for future rates, as they did in New York, the long-run incentive to cut costs is obviously weak, since greater efficiency this year translates into lower budgets in subsequent years.[125]

The fractions of hospital patients or revenues covered by the programs discussed in the second section are not overwhelming. For instance, the Rhode Island program applied only to Blue Cross patients, who accounted for but 40 percent of the state's total patient-days.[126] Similarly, the New Jersey program applied only to 43 percent of all inpatient-days. Coverage of the New York programs was not much greater; Medicare, commercially insured, and self-pay patients were excluded. Thus the limited scope of these programs may help to further explain their feeble impacts on costs.[127]

While the evidence of negative average-cost impacts in the rate-setting studies is weak, the evidence for negative total-cost impacts is even weaker because of possible positive effects on the volume of services. Several aspects of a rate-setting program may encourage volume increases. Volume-adjustment provisions that do not accurately distinguish marginal and average costs can encourage hospitals to exceed their volume projections.[128] In addition, incentives for high-volume projections may also exist.[129] For example, if relatively high unit costs increase the risk of cuts in proposed budgets during budget reviews, high-volume projections can be used to reduce this risk. Basing volume projections on actual volume in prior years also creates an incentive to increase actual volumes.[130] Finally, a volume-increasing incentive can be created through the appeals process if an unexpectedly large excess of actual over projected volume is acceptable grounds for renegotiating a prospectively determined budget.[131]

The research results have several implications for the effectiveness of rate setting in the future. The most optimistic view is that once the difficulties of the start-up period have been overcome, more substantial cost savings will be achieved, particularly if all patients are covered under rate setting. However, if efficiency incentives for hospitals under rate setting are indeed weak, then cost savings can be achieved only through stringent regulatory policies, with continuing conflict between rate setters and hospitals as a likely by-product. More attention to volume controls may be needed to counteract incentives to increase volumes. Detailed scrutiny of volume projections, and the use of utilization control procedures to restrict actual volume could be helpful. But in view of the current doubts about the effectiveness of utilization controls,[132] reliance on per case rates (rather than per diem or individual service rates) or limitations on total revenues may control use more effectively by diminishing incentives to increase volume.[133]

Clearly the effectiveness of rate setting depends on the behavior of regulators, and their behavior is influenced by the incentives and political pressures that confront them. The capture and political-economy theories imply that vigorous regulatory efforts to control costs are unlikely. But the empirical evidence for those theories as applied to hospital rate setting is less than overwhelming. There is a less pessimistic conceptualization of the influence of political pressures on regulatory behavior that seems intuitively more appealing. It has been suggested that regulators will respond to strong public pressure for resolving a particular problem but that once the problem has been brought under control and public pressure recedes, industry interests tend to dominate regulatory decision making.[134] This thesis raises the possibility that regulatory effectiveness will tend to vary cyclically or at least fluctuate over time. For example, when hospital costs are rising very rapidly and public concern is high, rate setters will adopt stringent control policies. As the rate of cost increase is slowed, which may not occur until operating procedures have been worked out during the start-up period, policies more favorable to hospital service expansion will result in an upsurge in inflation and a return to more stringent controls. The long-term prospect, according to this view, is for some improvement on average over the situation with no controls, but of a modest scale.

Of course, generalizations such as these have their dangers. These derive in part from the limitations and occasional technical deficiencies of the research. But more significant is that the estimates of rate-setting impacts apply to particular programs functioning within a complex political milieu in a limited period of time. The structures of these programs vary widely, the possibilities for restructuring are numerous, and the political climate varies from place to place and over time. Thus general statements about the likely effectiveness of rate-setting in all places and at all times must be regarded as speculative in the extreme.[135] This is particularly so at present because of the limited number of studies completed to date. One hopes that further research will help to establish a firmer basis for definitive policy conclusions.

Several suggestions about the nature of this further research are worthy of mention. First, if control of total health care costs remains the primary focus of policy, dependent variables should be chosen accordingly. Rather than emphasize average unit costs, researchers should pay more attention to rate-setting impacts on total hospital costs and on the costs of nonhospital services. Second, study periods that span a long experience with rate setting are needed to differentiate between start-up effects and the influence of mature programs. Third, new approaches to rate setting—such as per case reimbursement and total revenue limitation—need to be studied carefully, though experience with these mechanisms is limited at present. Fourth, with the proliferation of other types of regulation (especially PSROs and certificate-of-need), analysis of the joint effects of several different forms of controls are particularly relevant to current policy decisions.[136]

Finally, the general growth of cost-containment activities poses serious problems for future evaluation studies. Comparisons between appropriate control and experimental groups become more difficult as the spread of regulation reduces the available supply of control environments. The operation of national programs—such as the current voluntary cost-control effort sponsored by the American Hospital Association and other private organizations—makes it difficult to generalize the results of state-level studies to situations where those national programs are not operative or are configured differently from present programs. The frequent modifications of control programs to increase their effectiveness, coupled with uncertainty about the lags between these modifications and their full impact on costs, limits our ability to attribute research results to specific regulatory measures.[137] Perhaps this all implies that we should not expect too much in the way of clear answers from any one study and that it will be some time before a substantial stock of knowledge about the effectiveness of rate setting can be accumulated. In the meantime we shall have to follow Charles Lindblom's advice and simply "muddle through."[138]

Notes

1. Katherine G. Bauer, "Hospital Rate-Setting: This way to Salvation?" in *Hospital Cost Containment: Selected Notes for Future Policy*, ed. Michael Zubkoff, Ira E. Raskin, and Ruth S. Hanft (New York: Prodist, for the Milbank Memorial Fund, 1978), p. 325.

2. For detailed information on the specific procedures applied in various prospective rate-setting programs, see Bauer, "Hospital Rate Setting" and the references cited therein. Summary descriptions of several programs are also given in the second section of this chapter.

3. A review of several of these programs may be found in *Proposals for the Regulation of Hospital Costs* (Washington, D.C.: American Enterprise Institute, 1978).

4. The use of these different definitions of units of service is discussed at length in the literature on defining hospital output. See chapter 1 of this volume and Sylvester Berki, *Hospital Economics* (Lexington, Mass.: Lexington Books, D.C. Heath, 1972), chap. 2, for comparisons of the case and the day as measures of inpatient care output. Studies that emphasize specific outputs of departments within the hospital are William Dowling, *The Analysis of Hospital Production: A Linear Programming Approach* (Lexington, Mass.: Lexington Books, D.C. Heath, 1976) and Jeffrey Harris, "The Internal Organization of Hospitals: Some Economic Implications," *Bell Journal of Economics and Management Science* 8:(Autumn 1977) 467–482.

5. In this context excessive use could refer to productive inefficiency for the entire health care system. This would occur when services provided within hospitals could be provided at the same quality level and lower cost by nonhospital providers. Excessive use could also refer to allocative inefficiency—the marginal benefit of improved health of hospital care being too low to justify its marginal cost.

6. Roger Noll, "The Consequences of Public Utility Regulation of Hospitals," in Institute of Medicine, *Controls on Health Care* (Washington, D.C.: National Academy of Sciences, 1975).

7. U.S. Congress, Office of Technology Assessment, *Policy Implications of the Computed Tomography Scanner* (Washington, D.C.: U.S. Government Printing Office, 1978), chap 4; Chris Bale, "Is 'In and Out' Surgery Ready to Stay Put?" *Group Practice* (May-June 1977): 10–16, 34.

8. William L. Dowling, "Prospective Reimbursement of Hospitals," *Inquiry* 9 (September 1974): 163–180. This would reduce cost per day since the cost of each additional day is less than the average rost of earlier days in a hospital stay when treatment is more intensive.

9. Ibid.

10. Further discussion of this point may be found in David S. Sal-

kever and Alan Sorkin, "Economics and Health Economics," in *Health Services Administration Education, vol. 2: Behavioral and Social Sciences*, ed. Kent W. Peterson (Berkeley, Ca.: McCutchan Publishing Company, forthcoming).

11. A similar conclusion was expressed in recent papers by Berry and Chassin. See Ralph E. Berry, Jr., "Prospective Rate Regulation and Cost Containment: Formula Reimbursement in New York," *Inquiry* 13 (September 1976): 288–301, p. 299, and Mark B. Chassin, "The Containment of Hospital Costs: A Strategic Assessment," *Medical Care* 16 (October 1978): supplement, p. 45.

12. See Bauer, "Hospital Rate-Setting," p. 343.

13. Of course, PSROs and certificate-of-need programs are not meant to be solely concerned with limiting the quantity of services consumed. They are also intended to improve the quality of care and to assure that the health care system is responsive to community needs. Nevertheless, I think it fair to say that limitation of quantity (as a means of limiting total cost) has thus far been viewed as the most important goal of these programs.

14. See *Proposals for the Regulation of Hospital Costs*, pp. 17–20; Helen Thornberry and Harvey Zimmerman, *Hospital Cost Control: An Assessment of the Rhode Island Experience with Prospective Reimbursement, 1971 and 1972*, Final Report on Contract HEW-OS-74-197 (Providence, R.I.: Rhode Island Health Services Research, n.d.), pp. 294–299; Bauer, "Hospital Rate-Setting," p. 343; and Blue Cross Association, Maxicap Project Staff, "The Maxicap Primer" (Chicago, April 1978). Although policymakers may be concerned primarily with controlling total costs, they may not be indifferent between reductions in total costs that are achieved by reducing unit costs and reductions achieved by cuts in utilization. If reductions in unit cost represent pure efficiency gains while cuts in utilization eliminate services with positive marginal benefits (which may not outweigh their costs), the former will presumably be preferred. (I am indebted to Frank Sloan for this point.)

15. The term *experimental* is used here to signify areas or hospitals subject to rate-setting, while *control* shall mean the comparison areas in hospitals that are not subject to rate setting.

16. See the discussion of the Indiana rate-setting program in the second section of this chapter.

17. See Odin W. Anderson, *Health Care: Can There be Equity?* (New York: Wiley, 1972).

18. Another reason for being interested in these process measures of access is that they relate to the nonmonetary component of the cost of the health care system. This component is not included in available data on health care costs.

19. U.S. Department of Health, Education, and Welfare, Health Resources Administration, *Health United States, 1976–1977*, DHEW Publication (HRA) 77-1232, p. 21.

20. An example of the use of the impacts of insurance benefits in a related context is the analysis by Salkever and Bice of certificate-of-need regulation impacts on Medicare Part A and Part B benefit payments. See David S. Salkever and Thomas W. Bice, *Hospital Certificate-of-Need Controls: Impact on Investment Costs and Use* (Washington, D.C.: American Enterprise Institute, forthcoming), app. B.

21. Berry, "Prospective Rate Regulation," p. 299.

22. Another possible proxy for longer-term cost impacts is the effect of the rate-setting program on institutional changes in the health sector that are presumed to lead to lower costs, such as the growth of ambulatory surgery facilities, home care programs, and health maintenance organizations.

23. For references to the statistical literature on determinants of health levels see Joseph Newhouse and Lindy Friendlander, *The Relationship between Medical Resources and Measures of Health: Some Additional Evidence*, Rand Corporation Report R-2066-HEW (Santa Monica, Ca.:, May 1977); and Edward D. Colby, "Health Status and the Availability of Health Services System Resources" (Sc.D. thesis, Department of Medical Care and Hospitals, Johns Hopkins University, Baltimore, 1974), chap. 2.

24. Other approaches to measuring the quality of medical care emphasize either outcomes (results of treatment) or structure (the qualifications of the personnel providing care and the characteristics of other inputs into the care process). The former is generally regarded as conceptually preferable and does relate more directly to population health levels. However, the practical difficulties of carrying out outcome studies are formidable. For a discussion of various approaches to quality measurement, a basic reference is Avedis Donabedian, "Evaluating the Quality of Medical Care," *Milbank Memorial Fund Quarterly* 44 (July 1966): pp. 166–206.

25. This might not be viewed as an important criticism of the researchers who carried out the studies, however, given that their expertise lay primarily in the area of economics and not in quality assessment of medical practice.

26. Applied Management Sciences, *Analysis of Prospective Reimbursement Systems: Western Pennsylvania*, Final Report on Contract HEW-OS-74-226 (Silver Spring, Md.: August 6, 1975), chap. 3.

27. A sixth study completed under this research program (ibid.) evaluated a small-scale rate-setting experiment in Western Pennsylvania.

Since the experiment included only five hospitals and no econometric analyses were carried out in the study, it will not be discussed here.

28. See U.S. Department of Health, Education, and Welfare, Office of the Secretary, Request for Proposal No. 64-74-HEW-OS, January 2, 1974.

29. This description of the Rhode Island program is based on Thornberry and Zimmerman, *Hospital Cost Control*, chap. 4.

30. The program was not operative during fiscal 1973 and 1974 because of problems with the federal ESP controls.

31. This section is based on Geomet, *Analysis of the New Jersey Prospective Reimbursement System, 1968–1973*, Final Report on Contract HEW-OS-74-268 (Gaithersburg, Md., 1976), chap. 1.

32. Center for Analysis of Public Issues, *Bureaucratic Malpractice* (Princeton, N.J., 1974), chap. 1.

33. Material in this section was drawn from Abt Associates and Policy Analysis, *Analysis of Prospective Payment Systems for Upstate New York*, Final Report on Contract HEW-OS-74-261 (Cambridge, Mass., 1976), chap 2.

34. This description of the Indiana program is based on material in Spectrum Research, *Impact of the Indiana Prospective Payment Program on Hospitals*, Final Report on Contract HEW-OS-74-209 (Denver Colo., May 1978), chap. 3.

35. As such, it cannot legally compel hospitals to participate. But since Indiana Blue Cross enrollees make up 78 percent of the state population and the rates paid to nonparticipating hospitals are minimal, the hospital has strong financial incentives to participate in the rate-setting program. See ibid., pp. 3–4.

36. In several cases estimates were based only on before-and-after analyses of hospitals subject to rate setting.

37. The Rhode Island analysis excluded outpatient costs from the dependent variable while others included such costs and either included an independent variable for outpatient activity or adjusted the denominator of the dependent variable upward to reflect patient-day equivalents of outpatient visits.

38. The symbol ˆ denotes an estimated value for a coefficient.

39. See table 4–1. Total cost was also used as a dependent variable in the upstate New York study. Abt Associates and Policy Analysis, *Analysis of Prospective Payment Systems for Upstate New York*, chap. 7.

40. Ibid.

41. For examples of quasi-technological cost functions, see chapter 1 of this volume. Chapter 2 specifies and estimates behavioral cost equations.

42. The recognition that explanatory variables measuring capital stock and output may be influenced by rate setting points up another potential problem, namely, simultaneous equation bias. One suspects that this problem is more serious in the quasi-technological approach, since more endogenous variables are used as regressors.

43. One might, of course, justify any number of additional variables in a quasi-technological cost function on the grounds that they influence product quality or hospital efficiency. However, as the number of additional variables increases, this rationale becomes less persuasive.

44. Geomet, *Analysis of the New Jersey Prospective Reimbursement Program*, chap. 3.

45. Geomet also estimated a number of linear equations in which the dependent variable was defined as the year-to-year change in average cost per day (case) and independent variables included changes in the occupancy (case-flow) rate and the number of days (admissions), the lagged value of average cost per day (case), and a rate-setting dummy. This model implies that rate setting will have an effect on the relative rate of cost increase which is constant over time. However, the conceptual basis of this model is unclear. Lagged cost variables have been used in behavioral models to reflect partial adjustment processes, but this interpretation seems rather odd for quasi-technological cost functions.

46. Ginsburg, for example, has suggested using separate rate-setting dummies for hospitals entering the New Jersey program in different years. Since the hospitals entering the program in earlier years had higher costs, one might expect a greater rate-setting effect on these hospitals. See Paul B. Ginsburg, *Reform in the Reimbursement of Health Care Institutions* (Washington, D.C.: American Enterprise Institute, forthcoming), chap. 4.

47. It is surprising that Hellinger's report on the New Jersey experiment makes no reference to the rather discouraging results of the Geomet cost analysis. Instead he presents a single regression specification using data from New Jersey hospitals for 1969–1973. His dependent variable is average cost (per day or per case), and his explanatory variables include a lagged dependent variable and some of the other independent variables used in the Geomet analysis. While he applies ordinary least squares and obtains a negative rate-setting coefficient in his cost-per-day equation with a t-value of 1.001, the corresponding coefficient in his cost-per-case regression is positive. In view of potential econometric problems due to the lagged dependent variable, the difficulty of interpreting this type of regression specification, and the consistently poor Geomet results, the insignificantly negative rate-setting coefficient in Helliner's cost-per-day equation obviously does not alter the pessimistic conclusion. See Fred J. Hellinger, "An Empirical Analysis of Several Prospective Reimburse-

ment Systems,'' in *Hospital Cost Containment*, ed. Zubkoff, Raskin, and Hanft, pp. 370–400.

48. Thornberry and Zimmerman, *Hospital Cost Control*, chap. 5.

49. Thornberry and Zimmerman considered this procedure but rejected it because F-tests on Rhode Island and Massachusetts data for 1969–1970 indicated significant differences in cost-function coefficients between the states. In view of the resulting methodological difficulties, the wisdom of this decision may be questioned. Moreover, it is conceivable that simply including separate intercepts for each state in the 1969–1970 analysis would have reversed the result of the F-test. Unfortunately, it is difficult to assess this conjecture, since the relevant regression results were not reported.

50. This calculation ignores the possible effect of the program on endogenous explanatory variables such as the occupancy rate and length of stay. I return to this point in the second section of this chapter.

51. Lester P. Silverman, ''The Effect of Prospective Reimbursement on Cost in Rhode Island Hospitals,'' Center for Naval Analysis, February 1975. This paper appears as Attachment F in Thornberry and Zimmerman, *Hospital Cost Control*.

52. These cost functions differed only slightly from the linear functions estimated by Thornberry and Zimmerman. Silverman included a separate dummy for 1970 and did not deflate his dependent variable by a cost index. He also deleted the least significant of the case-mix variables from the analysis and aggregated the remaining case-mix variables into four groupings (based on similarity of their initial coefficient estimates).

53. Abt Associates and Policy Analysis, *Analysis of Prospective Payment Systems for Upstate New York*, chap. 5.

54. Ibid., p. V-22.

55. This is equivalent to assuming $\gamma_1 \text{-} \gamma_2 \text{-} \gamma_3 = \gamma_4 = 0$ in equation 4.4.

56. This is obvious once it is recalled that all the γ's are linear combinations of the same vector of random variables (the regression disturbances). For an example of mutually exclusive dummy variables and nonzero covariances between their coefficients, see David S. Salkever, ''The Use of Dummy Variables to Compute Predictions, Prediction Errors, and Confidence Intervals,'' *Journal of Econometrics* 4 (November 1976):393–397.

57. It is rather odd that these technical errors do not recur in Abt's analysis of rate-setting effects on hospital production functions, since the overall design of the cost and production function analyses are the same. Apparently there was a lack of communication between the different researchers conducting these two analyses.

58. These effects cannot actually be computed because the report does not indicate exactly how the time-trend variables are coded.

59. William L. Dowling et al., *The Impact of the Blue Cross and Medicaid Prospective Reimbursement Systems in Downstate New York*, Final Report on Contract HEW-OS-74-248, Department of Health Services, School of Public Health and Community Medicine, University of Washington (Seattle, June 1976). Estimated cost functions are described in chapter 5 of the report, and the process of control-group selection is explained in chapter 2.

60. The wage components of the price indexes were based on reported hospital wages rather than on data from other sectors. If the downstate New York rate-setting program slowed the rise in wages, the effect of this slowdown on cost would be largely controlled for through the deflation procedure and would not appear in the regression estimates of rate-setting effects. For discussion of rate-setting effects on wages, see the second section of this chapter.

61. The use of separate equations for each area was based on F-tests that indicated significant differences in regression coefficients among the areas.

62. However, all the independent variables except admissions, patient-days, and occupancy entered the log-linear regressions in linear form.

63. It is not possible to determine significance levels for the differences in intercept shifts or for total rate-setting effects because covariances of the coefficient estimates are not reported.

64. See Dowling et al., *Impact of Prospective Reimbursement in Downstate New York*, chap. 1.

65. It is not clear whether a single regression was estimated or two separate regressions were run (for experimental hospitals and for all control hospitals combined).

66. Similarly, it is not possible to compute the magnitude and significance of the total rate-setting effect. In other regressions presented by Dowling et al., the rate-setting variable is defined as the percentage of patients or revenues covered under the rate-setting program. However, these regressions included only experimental hospitals and their results were not used to compute rate-setting effects. For some reason this method of specifying a rate-setting variable was not employed in any of the analyses described in the text.

67. Hellinger, "An Empirical Analysis of Several Prospective Reimbursement Systems," pp. 388–402.

68. It is unfortunate that Hellinger does not refer to any of the results presented in the downstate New York report. Thus the particular reasons for his more significant findings are not clear.

69. The methods and results of this study are presented in Spectrum Research, *Impact of the Indiana Program*, chap. 13–22.

70. The total effect of rate setting is the difference between actual cost levels in Indiana hospitals and the levels that would have been observed if the rate-setting program had never been implemented.

71. In most cases Michigan Blue Cross actually relied on local planning agency project reviews. The principal focus of these reviews appears to have been construction of new hospitals and expansion of bed supplies rather than investment in new equipment or services (see Spectrum Research, *Impact of the Indiana Program*, chap. 13).

72. The conceptual model of hospital behavior is presented and discussed in ibid., chap. 14 and app. A.

73. This may be a difficult task, however, if the model takes account of strategic interactions between hospital and regulator behavior.

74. Strictly speaking, of course, no state is entirely free from hospital regulation if regulation is defined to include licensing provisions and regulation of health insurance premiums. Thus the difference between Michigan and Spectrum's other control states is a matter of degree. Moreover, this difference depends on the effectiveness of Michigan's capital-expenditure review program.

75. Published data on wage rates only partially confirm this speculation. Data from *County Business Patterns* (U.S. Department of Commerce) show that average payroll per employee in the service industries increased by only 34.8 percent in Indiana over the 1968–1973 period while increases in control states ranged from 35.2 percent (Iowa) to 42.2 percent (Minnesota). On the other hand, data on hourly earnings in manufacturing from the *Handbook of Labor Statistics* (U.S. Department of Labor) show an increase of 39.6 percent for Indiana over this period while control state increases ranged from 34.5 percent (Minnesota) to 39.4 percent (Iowa).

76. The percentage increases cited here are based on *Guide Issue* data for all nonfederal short-term general and other hospitals.

77. The fact that Spectrum obtained larger estimated program impacts with the Michigan control group than with the Illinois-Iowa-Minnesota control group supports this observation. However, the figures cited in the text are for all hospitals while Spectrum's analysis was restricted to control hospitals selected to match the characteristics of the Indiana hospitals.

78. For a discussion of these methods see Yair Mundlak, "On the Pooling of Time Series and Cross-Section Data," Harvard Institute of Economic Research Discussion Paper 457 (Cambridge, Mass., February 1976).

79. The New Jersey study does not present any evidence pertaining to these matters.

80. Other types of effects—relating to administrative practices, input mix, production functions, and costs and productivity in particular de-

partments (or groups of departments)—were also studied but will not be discussed here.

81. The comparisons are presented in Silverman, "The Effect of Prospective Reinbursement."

82. Additional trend data for Rhode Island on admissions, case-mix, and other variables are presented in Thornberry and Zimmerman, *Hospital Cost Control*, chaps. 6 and 8. However, comparable control-group data are not shown and thus it is not possible to distinguish Rhode Island program effects from the effects of federal price controls.

83. See Abt Associates and Policy Analysis, *Analysis of Prospective Payment Systems for Upstate New York*, chap. 5.

84. However, if these effects were based on regression analyses similar to Abt's cost regressions, the previously noted problems with their calculations of effects and associated standard errors presumably apply. The Abt report (chap. 6) also presents regression analyses of beds, admissions, occupancy, and length of stay based on data for experimental hospitals for the years 1970–1974. The rate-setting variables in these regressions include the percentages of patient-days to which rates were applicable (the percentages accounted for by Blue Cross and Medicaid beneficiaries) and the extent to which hospitals incurred various penalties under the program. While the results of these analyses are quite mixed, they provide some support for the hypothesis that hospitals increase length of stay and occupancy rate to mitigate the effect of tight per diem rates. Of course, the force of this conclusion is weakened by the absence of control-group hospitals in the analyses.

85. Quality-enhancing services and facilities include the most commonly found items, such as postoperative recovery rooms and emergency departments. Complexity-enhancing items relate to more sophisticated treatment procedures. Examples are burn care units, renal dialysis, intensive care, open heart surgery, and therapeutic radiology facilities. Community services include social work, family planning, home care, extended care, rehabilitation services, outpatient services, and self-care units.

86. More generally, the validity of these regression results is questionable because of econometric problems involved in using ordinary least squares with a lagged dependent variable. See for example, Jan Kmenta, *Elements of Econometrics* (New York: Macmillan, 1971), chap. 11. Other scope-of-service regressions in chapter 11 of the Abt report were carried out separately for large hospitals (> 200 beds) and for small hospitals (< 200 beds). While these indicate that rate setting may have slowed the growth of complexity-expanding services among small hospitals, the inclusion of lagged dependent variables again poses problems.

87. The 1968–1974 increase in the CPI for the New York metropoli-

tan area was 48.3 percent. The corresponding figures for Philadelphia, Chicago, and Cleveland were 44.7 percent, 40.1 percent, and 39.6 percent respectively.

88. Some back-of-the-envelope calculations in chapter 1 of the downstate New York report indicate that perhaps as much as 70 percent of these savings were offset by volume increases due to rate setting.

89. A regression analysis of length of stay, based on 1968–1974 data for experimental hospitals, was also presented in chapter 6 of the downstate New York report. The rate-setting variable in this analysis (percentage of revenues under rate controls) had a positive but insignificant effect.

90. These measures were (1) the overall average length of stay, (2) a case-mix-adjusted length-of-stay index for diagnostic categories in which case severity was thought to be the primary determinant of length of stay, and (3) a similar index for diagnostic categories in which physician behavior was thought to be the primary determinant of length of stay.

91. See chapters 23, 26, and 31 of the Spectrum report.

92. See, for example, Salkever and Bice, *Hospital Certificate-of-Need Controls*, chap 4, and the references cited there.

93. The upstate New York report presents comparative data on nonaccredited hospitals (chap. 10). But since the percentage of nonaccredited hospitals is generally quite low, it is not too surprising that no clear difference between experimental and control groups was found.

94. The New Jersey study did not examine financial impacts.

95. The relevant regressions are reported in table D-9 of the Abt report. Unfortunately, the significance of this effect could not be determined precisely because of the problems in Abt's methods for computing rate-setting effects and standard errors.

96. See chapter 7 of the downstate New York report for a definition of these terms.

97. A recent reanalysis of the downstate New York data by Urban yields similar results. Using regression techniques, she fails to find consistently negative rate-setting effects on profitability and liquidity. See Nicole Urban, "A Summary of the Impact of Prospective Reimbursement on Hospital Financial Position in Downstate New York," Discussion Paper 10, Health Policy Research Series, Department of Health Services, University of Washington, Seattle, August 1978.

98. Another interpretation of the insignificance of rate-setting effects is given in the Abt report (p. V-29). (See also Jerry Cromwell et al., "An Analysis of Prospective Payment Systems in Upstate New York," Discussion Paper HCSA-3, Abt Associates, Cambridge, Mass., November 1976.) It is asserted there that the negative estimated rate-setting effects show *"what actually happened on average"* (emphasis in original) while

the insignificance of those effects indicates that they should not be generalized to other time periods, other groups of hospitals, or other geographic areas. Of course, this assertion is wrong, since it would imply that any explanatory variable (for example, the won-lost record of the New York Mets) actually influenced the level of costs except in the highly unlikely case where its coefficient was exactly zero.

99. The description of the ESP presented here is based primarily on Ginsburg, *Reform in the Reimbursement of Health Care Institutions*, chap. 3, and "Inflation and the Economic Stabilization Program," in *Health: A Victim or Cause of Inflation?* ed. M. Zubkoff (New York: Prodist, for the Milbank Memorial Fund, 1976), pp. 31–51.

100. During the period November 14 to December 30, 1971, the regulations for all service industries were applicable to hospitals.

101. The 6 percent figure included a 1.7 percent increment for new technology. However, the definition of expenses that could be classified under the new technology provision was limited; thus for many hospitals the effective constraint on price increases was 4.3 percent.

102. For the details of both volume indexes, see Ginsburg, "Inflation and the Economic Stabilization Program," pp. 41–43.

103. Joseph Lipscomb, Ira Raskin, and Joseph Eichenholz, "The Use of Hospital Cost Estimates in Hospital Cost Containment Policy," in *Hospital Cost Containment*, ed. Zubkoff, Raskin, and Hanft pp. 514–537.

104. Phase III of the ESP, which began in January 1973, replaced the phase II mandatory controls with voluntary guidelines in most sectors. But the mandatory Phase II controls for health services were continued during this period. See Touche Ross & Co., *Economic Stabilization Program* (1973), p. 1.

105. The proposed Phase IV regulations are discussed in Stuart Altman and Joseph Eichenholz, "Inflation in the Health Care Industry: Causes and Cures," in *Health: A Victim or Cause of Inflation?* ed. Zubkoff, pp. 7–30.

106. Paul B. Ginsburg, "Impact of the Economic Stabilization Program on Hospitals: An Analysis with Aggregate Data," in *Hospital Cost Containment*, ed. Zubkoff, Raskin, and Hanft, pp. 293–323.

107. This procedure yields estimated ESP effects that do not include any possible ESP influence on length of stay.

108. Frank A. Sloan and Bruce Steinwald, "Effects of Regulation on Hospital Costs and Inpatient Use" (paper presented at the Annual Meeting of the American Economic Association, Chicago, August 29, 1978). Sloan and Steinwald estimate effects of both the ESP and a variety of other control programs though only the former are discussed here.

109. These variables were selected on the basis of a model of hospital

behavior similar to that used by Ginsburg. With a lagged dependent variable included, the model implies that observed hospital behavior represents a proportional adjustment toward an equilibrium situation. However, the addition of regulatory variables strains this interpretation somewhat. While it implies that regulation shifts the equilibrium position, it also reflects the convenient but curious assumption that the hospital-regulator adjustment process to equilibrium is the same as the hospital adjustment process in the absence of regulation.

110. Those with lagged dependent variables were estimated with a technique developed by Nerlove for pooled data. (See Marc Nerlove, "Further Evidence on the Estimation of Dynamic Economic Relations from a Time Series of Cross Sections," *Econometrica* 39(1971):359–382.) Those without lagged variables were estimated by ordinary least squares. In the latter case the presence of hospital-specific error components may result in underestimates of coefficient standard errors. For a discussion of the limitations of the Nerlove procedure, see Mundlak, "On the Pooling of Time-Series and Cross-Section Data."

111. A possible explanation is that wage increases of low-wage workers were not subject to controls, since hospital wages tend to be low relative to those in other industries. But while increased wages of low-paid workers could be used as grounds for an exception, the fact that exceptions were usually not granted unless hospitals had a negative cash flow may have discouraged liberal wage increases. See Ginsburg, *Reform in the Reimbursement of Health Care Institutions*, chap 3, for further discussion of this point.

112. For example, Ginsburg included time-trend and CPI variables in his equations and used undeflated data while Sloan and Steinwald excluded these variables and used deflated data.

113. Salkever and Bice, *Hospital Certificate-of-Need Controls*, chap 5.

114. Martin Feldstein, "Quality Change and the Demand for Hospital Care," *Econometrica* 45 (1977):1681–1702.

115. Judith R. Lave and Lester B. Lave, "Hospital Cost Function Analysis: Implications for Cost Controls," in *Hospital Cost Containment*, ed. Zubkoff, Raskin, and Hanft, pp. 538–571.

116. Though both these specifications avoid the omitted case-mix variable problem, they have their disadvantages. Their implied expressions for marginal cost in any year are quite complicated and involve values of the explanatory variables for a number of different years. Also they imply that random influences on cost in any one year affect the dependent variable values in two or more years, so the possibility of autocorrelation must be considered. Other approaches that avoid these

difficulties (but are more cumbersome to implement) are the inclusion of separate intercepts for each hospital and the use of first-differenced data and generalized least squares (to correct for autocorrelation).

117. In this connection, table 4–3 indicates a marked drop in cost inflation over the 1973–1974 period.

118. On the other hand, the fact that the rate of cost inflation surged in late 1974 after the lapse of controls argues against this conjecture. See "Hospital Indicators," *Hospitals* 49:21–28.

119. The most extreme example of this is the ESP. See Ginsburg, "Inflation and the Economic Stabilization Program."

120. In addition, stopgap measures during the pre-rate-setting years may have diminished pre–post differences. An example is the freeze on Medicaid hospital rates in New York adopted in March 1969. See Abt Associates and Policy Analysis, *Analysis of Prospective Payment Systems for Upstate New York*, chap. 2.

121. With the continued growth of the hospital labor force, the political pressures against stringent cost controls will grow. This point is made forcefully by Louise B. Russell, "Medical Care Costs," in *Setting National Priorities: The 1978 Budget*, ed. Joseph A. Pechman (Washington, D.C.: Brookings Institution, 1977), pp. 177–206.

122. The capture and political economy theories are described more fully in Noll, "The Consequences of Public Utility Regulation of Hospitals."

123. The fact that the state program that appears to have been the most effective (Indiana) worked closely with hospital representatives runs counter to the capture theory.

124. This incentive did not exist in the New Jersey program because reimbursements were limited to actual costs when costs were below the prospectively determined rates.

125. See Bauer, "Hospital Rate-Setting," p. 359. This is a familiar point in the public utility literature. Regulatory lags in adjusting rates to observed costs create efficiency incentives.

126. Thornberry and Zimmerman, *Hospital Cost Control*, Attachment F.

127. While the coverage of the Indiana program was limited to Blue Cross beneficiaries, the program effectively discouraged the hospitals from using different rates for other patient groups.

128. Volume-adjustment provisions are formulas used to change hospital rates automatically when actual volume deviates from projected volume. Penalties for failure to achieve minimum occupancy rates provide incentives for increased volume.

129. Bauer, "Hospital Rate-Setting," p. 351.

130. At the same time there may be a disincentive to high-volume

projections. They may reduce the short-run opportunities for earning net revenues that exist under a volume-adjustment system that overstates the ratio of marginal to average costs.

131. This was the case, for example, in the Rhode Island program.

132. For a brief review of the evidence and further references, see David S. Salkever, "Will Regulation Control Hospital Costs," *Bulletin of the New York Academy of Medicine* 54(1978):73–83.

133. It is generally assumed that admission rates are less susceptible than length of stay to control by the hospital. Furthermore, per case rates create incentives to reduce length of stay even though they may also increase the number of admissions.

134. See Barry R. Weingast, "A Positive Model of Public Policy Formation: The Case of Regulatory Agency Behavior," Center for the Study of American Business Working Paper 25, Washington University, St. Louis, January 1978.

135. The variation in results reported in the second section gives further reason to treat such general statements cautiously.

136. Studies that examine these joint effects should not assume that the effect of the controls are simply additive, since they may tend to reinforce one another in producing desired results or undesired side effects. In this connection, it would be interesting to see what results the Sloan-Steinwald analysis would yield if interactions for utilization review, rate setting, and certificate-of-need programs were included.

137. A more extensive discussion of these and other methodological problems is found in Ginsburg, *Reform in the Reimbursement of Health Case Institutions*, chaps. 3, 4.

138. Charles E. Lindblom, "The Science of 'Muddling Through,'" *Public Administration Review* 19(1959):79–88.

Index

About the Author

David S. Salkever is associate professor of health services administration at The Johns Hopkins School of Hygiene and Public Health. He received the Ph.D. in economics from Harvard University in 1970. Dr. Salkever is the author of numerous articles dealing with hospital costs and their regulation and is coauthor (with Thomas W. Bice) of *Hospital Certificate-of-Need Controls* (American Enterprise Institute for Public Policy Research, forthcoming).